"This book will certainly get you and your staff talking; it provides a truly accessible blend of theory and practice to enable practitioners to recognise that all-inclusive environments need a strong emphasis on speech, language and communication. It offers a timely contribution to the sector, recognising the need to focus on oracy and putting these skills firmly at the core of the curriculum."

— **Diana Bannister MBE**, *Professor, University of Wolverhampton, UK.*

"I am thrilled to see time and space being given to a key area of development that is so often overlooked or simply taken for granted. My time with I CAN taught me just how vital a child's ability to communicate was to their future life chances, and my own research with schools proved the inextricable link between communication skills and a child's confidence, independence and general wellbeing. Understanding ways to support communication is vital for every educator—in all stages of education—every teacher should read this book."

—**Carla Solvason**, *University of Worcester, UK.*

"*Developing Speech, Language and Communication Skills in Education: What Works and Why*? neatly interweaves research and practice. It explores a range of speech, language and communication factors from different author perspectives, reflecting on current Speech and Language Therapy from a fresh and forward-thinking perspective. I recommend this title to all SaLTs who work in education."

—**Stephen Parsons** *@WordAware, UK.*

Developing Speech, Language, and Communication Skills in Education

This practical guide equips teachers, educators, and speech and language therapists who work across the age phases with the knowledge, skills, and confidence required to fully meet the speech, language, and communication (SLC) needs of children and young people (CYP). As SLC challenges are increasing among pupils, this book links theory to practical aspects of pedagogy, guiding readers to consider how to support the CYP they work with in educational settings. It champions a collaborative approach to supporting conditions such as Developmental Language Disorder (DLD), Autism, and others, and considers the reasonable adjustments that can be implemented to support all pupils (a 'universal' approach). Written by a multi-disciplinary team, it embraces sociological, educational, and medical perspectives, encouraging critical thinking and offering a range of case studies that illustrate key strategies and real-world applications, as well as signposting practical resources and sources of further support.

Hazel Richards is a specialist speech and language therapist who worked with children and young people with complex needs in mainstream, specialist, and alternative settings for over 20 years. Her experience of working with SENCos as a professional, school governor, and parent motivated her doctoral studies investigating SENCo identity and influences on practice.

Natacha Capener has over 16 years' experience working within education, from early years through to secondary, in both mainstream and specialist settings. As a speech and language therapist she has worked collaboratively with teaching staff in schools to embed speech and language therapy practices and approaches within the academic curriculum.

Aaron Emmett is a speech and language therapist whose most recent clinical role was lead for secondary and further education. He has worked with children and young people as part of a secondary school team and as a youth worker. Aaron has engaged in research analysing the experiences of SENCos in accessing speech and language therapy services.

Developing Speech, Language, and Communication Skills in Education

What Works and Why

Edited by
Hazel Richards, Natacha Capener,
and Aaron Emmett

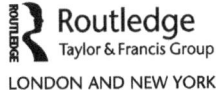

Routledge
Taylor & Francis Group
LONDON AND NEW YORK

Designed cover image: Critical Publishing

First published 2026
by Routledge
4 Park Square, Milton Park, Abingdon, Oxon OX14 4RN

and by Routledge
605 Third Avenue, New York, NY 10158

Routledge is an imprint of the Taylor & Francis Group, an informa business

© 2026 selection and editorial matter, Hazel Richards, Natacha Capener and Aaron Emmett; individual chapters, the contributors

The right of Hazel Richards, Natacha Capener and Aaron Emmett to be identified as the authors of the editorial material, and of the authors for their individual chapters, has been asserted in accordance with sections 77 and 78 of the Copyright, Designs and Patents Act 1988.

All rights reserved. No part of this book may be reprinted or reproduced or utilised in any form or by any electronic, mechanical, or other means, now known or hereafter invented, including photocopying and recording, or in any information storage or retrieval system, without permission in writing from the publishers.

For Product Safety Concerns and Information please contact our EU representative GPSR@taylorandfrancis.com. Taylor & Francis Verlag GmbH, Kaufingerstraße 24, 80331 München, Germany.

Trademark notice: Product or corporate names may be trademarks or registered trademarks, and are used only for identification and explanation without intent to infringe.

British Library Cataloguing-in-Publication Data
A catalogue record for this book is available from the British Library

ISBN: 978-1-041-05499-3 (hbk)
ISBN: 978-1-916-92581-6 (pbk)
ISBN: 978-1-041-05498-6 (ebk)

DOI: 10.4324/9781041054986

Typeset in ITC Franklin Gothic
by SPi Technologies India Pvt Ltd (Straive)

For Calum – who showed me speech language and communication development in real time and taught me SO much.
Hazel

For all the inspirational young people I have worked with. I've learned more from you than you ever did from me.
Aaron

For my wonderful family and the fantastic children, young people, and colleagues I have worked with over the years – couldn't have done it without you.
Natacha

Contents

Acknowledgements xi

Notes on the editors xii

Notes on the contributors xiii

Glossary of terms and abbreviations xv

Introduction 1

SECTION I: FUNDAMENTALS 7

1 Inclusive pedagogy for supporting speech, language and communication 9
STEPHANIE BREWSTER

2 Attention and listening 23
HAZEL RICHARDS

3 Play and conceptual development 39
TOM HOPKINS

4 Emotional regulation in the classroom 52
HELEN KNOWLER

5 Multilingualism: Growing up with more than one language 65
AYDAN SUPHI

SECTION II: KEY SPEECH, LANGUAGE, AND COMMUNICATION AREAS 77

6 Speech 79
CHARLIE AYLING AND LORRAINE BAMBLETT

7 Understanding and using language 92
LORRAINE BAMBLETT AND NATACHA CAPENER

8	Literacy and language TOM HOPKINS AND NATACHA CAPENER	107
9	Communication intent and social interaction HAZEL RICHARDS	124
10	Enabling communication for children who stammer AARON EMMETT	141
11	Supporting the communication of children and young people with social, emotional and mental health (SEMH) needs CLAIRE WESTWOOD AND TERI OAKSHOTT-MARSTON	153
12	Speech, language and communication needs in the school exclusion process CLAIRE WESTWOOD AND HELEN KNOWLER	167

SECTION III: IMPLEMENTATION AND MOVING FORWARD — 183

13	Preparation for adulthood AARON EMMETT	185
14	Creating inclusive environments that maximise functional speech, language and communication skills NIKI STOKES AND LORRAINE BAMBLETT	197
15	Interprofessional and collaborative working SALLY PHILPOTTS AND ALICE MURPHY	211
	Conclusion	226
	Index	228

Acknowledgements

We are indebted to the many people who gave generously of their time and expertise to produce this book. First, we would like to acknowledge the contribution of all the authors who delivered timely and well-researched chapters. Their professionalism and willingness to meet deadlines and respond to the comments of the reviewers, especially when all hold considerable workloads, made editing this book a pleasure.

Particular thanks go to the teachers and colleagues who provided the case studies which do so much to apply and bring the chapter material to life.

Thanks also go to our respective families and friends, who have provided much needed moral support, understanding and encouragement throughout.

We would like to acknowledge the generosity of:

- Mary Doherty, Sue McCown and Sebastian Shaw for permission to use the Autistic SPACE framework (reproduced with kind permission from the authors in Chapter 9);
- © Widgit Software Ltd. 2002–2025 for their permission, granted by Anna Cawrey, Partnerships Manager, Widgit, March 2025, to include Widgit Symbols in the resources shown in Chapters 7 and 13;
- RAND, for permission to use an adaptation of Catherine Snow's (2002) heuristic for thinking about reading comprehension https://www.rand.org/pubs/monograph_reports/MR1465.html. In Chapter 8.
- Spotlight, reading images: Flaticon.com. These images have been designed using resources from Flaticon.com.

We would also like to thank the Department of Speech and Language Therapy, Faculty of Health, Education and Life Sciences, Birmingham City University, where many of us work.

We would like to thank Julia Morris at Critical Publishing and Annamarie Kino at Taylor and Francis who have provided wise and responsive guidance throughout the process, as well as colleagues in the field who reviewed and critiqued the book at various stages of development.

Finally, we would like to thank the children and young people and their families who continue to inspire us with their determination, resilience and wonderful uniqueness.

Notes on the editors

Hazel Richards is a speech and language therapist who worked primarily in mainstream and specialist educational settings, before completing an MA in special and inclusive education. She left the NHS to teach education studies and SEND modules at undergraduate and master's level. On completing her PhD, which investigated an area of SENCo practice, she became a senior lecturer in Child and Family Studies, then trained SENCos at the universities of Worcester and Wolverhampton. She currently works at Birmingham City University, with undergraduate (traditional and degree apprentice routes) and post-graduate speech and language therapy students, including those conducting research. This allows her to combine her passions for equipping future professionals and empowering the voice and agency of clients experiencing speech, language and communication difficulties. A common thread throughout her career has been bridging health and education by recognising and harnessing the skills and knowledge of each to develop practice in both.

Aaron Emmett is a speech and language therapist who has worked with children and young people with SLCN for over a decade. Before taking his current post as a lecturer in speech and language therapy at Birmingham City University, his role was in the NHS as a highly specialist SaLT with older children and adolescents where he worked extensively with teenagers with language disorders and children and young people who stammer. Aaron's areas of teaching and research interest are around joint working with secondary schools and further education institutions to meet the needs of young adults with communication difficulties.

Natacha Capener is a speech and language therapist and lecturer. She graduated from University College London with an MSc in Speech and Language Sciences in 2012. Throughout her career she has worked in a range of mainstream and specialist schools, working with children and young people across the age span who have a range of language and communication challenges. She has worked in the NHS and as a direct employee of schools, in both 'traditional' and consultancy roles. She is passionate about collaboration and her area of specialism is in working with others to embed speech and language therapy approaches within curricula and school settings. She jointly set up the Birmingham Special Schools SaLT Network which provides peer supervision and skill sharing for SaLTs and communication specialists who are directly employed in educational settings across the city.

Notes on the contributors

Charlie Ayling is a lecturer in speech and language therapy at Birmingham City University and a speech and language therapist (SaLT) specialising in speech sound disorders (SSD) working for Birmingham Community NHS Foundation Trust. Charlie has worked with children in mainstream school settings and community clinics for over a decade, developing a specific interest and depth of experience in SSD over this time. She completed a master's in speech sound difficulties in 2022 and provides training and support to speech and language therapists and education staff working with children with SSD.

Lorraine Bamblett is a speech and language therapist who has worked in community clinics, Sure Start children's centres, pupil referral units, and mainstream and special schools, becoming a Specialist SaLT in 2008 within an enhanced resource for children with speech sound disorders, developmental language disorder and social communication needs. Lorraine has taught at Birmingham City University from 2021 to 2025 and now at Keele University. Lorraine has a master's in clinical research. Her areas of specialism are speech sound disorders, phonetics, telehealth and Developmental Language Disorder and she is a co-author of the 2024 Royal College of Speech and Language Therapists clinical guidance for Speech Sound Disorders.

Stephanie Brewster started out as a speech and language therapist working with a wide range of children and adults with communication needs. On completing a doctorate in education, she moved into higher education. Engaged in teaching and research in many areas of disability and diversity, she is a senior lecturer at the University of Wolverhampton, working with undergraduate and post-graduate learners, including those undergoing continuing professional development and conducting research. The common thread throughout her career is a concern with issues of exclusion, marginalisation and disadvantage, and how policy and practice can address these.

Tom Hopkins is a senior lecturer in speech and language therapy at Birmingham City University, teaching in areas of psychology and child development, including language and literacy development. Tom's background is in psychology, especially areas related to developmental and forensic psychology, with an interest in exploring the association between language, literacy and offending behaviour. Tom has worked on funded research projects that have identified language and literacy difficulties in children and young people considered 'at risk'. His published research also involves examining interventions that support language and literacy abilities in children, young people and adults.

Helen Knowler is a qualified teacher who has worked in the field of SEMH needs for over three decades. She became a higher education lecturer in 2006 and has worked at the universities of Plymouth, Bristol, Exeter and Wolverhampton. She now leads the Eugenics Legacy Education Project at University College London (UCL). Helen's expertise relates to school exclusion and specifically illegal and hidden exclusion and she is deeply committed to social justice in both her teaching and research. She has published widely in academic journals including the *British Journal of Special Education*, *Support for Learning* and *Journal of Research in Special Educational Needs*.

Alice Murphy is a qualified speech and language therapist with extensive experience working with children and young people with special educational needs, particularly those with social, emotional and mental health needs within Birmingham and the Black Country. Alice is passionate about supporting children and colleagues directly in her role as well as campaigning for wider systemic change; this has included being involved in local and national campaigns, presenting within a national webinar, and offering training to magistrates.

Teri Oakshott-Marston is an associate assistant headteacher and SENDCo at a medical and mental health alternative provision in the West Midlands. She graduated with a BA (Hons) in English Literature with English Language Studies from Birmingham City University in 2008 before beginning her teaching career with a PGCE in English from Newman University College in 2010. Teri has taught and led on SEND across primary and secondary mainstream settings, having completed NASENCO in 2014. Teri delivers outreach work and training as part of her role and continues to have a passion for inclusive practice in all school settings.

Sally Philpotts has worked in education since 2007, holding various curriculum and pastoral leadership roles within this time. Sally has previously worked as a Multi-Academy Trust (MAT) Director of SEND, collaborating with SENCos from 12 primary and secondary schools, enhancing systems and processes to promote inclusive provision. Sally is currently working as a MAT director of inclusion, focusing on the importance of supporting students holistically – recognising that academic success is deeply intertwined with emotional and social wellbeing.

Niki Stokes graduated with BA (Hons) in Interdisciplinary Human Studies from the University of Bradford in 1995, completed a post-graduate certificate at Liverpool University, and worked in marketing, PR, the music industry and publishing. A 2002 career break after starting a family led to involvement with Sure Start in North London, teaching Sing & Sign and supporting new mums. Niki completed a PGCE (Early Years) in 2009 after volunteering in pre-school governance. She has worked in mainstream Early Years settings, including in enhanced resources for pupils with speech, language and communication needs, SEMH and autism. As SENDCO, Niki completed the NASENCO in 2023.

Claire Westwood is a speech and language therapist with over a decade of experience in youth justice, school exclusions and mental health, aiming to block the school-to-prison pipeline via equitable communication access. Claire has worked as a university lecturer, court intermediary and currently is a designated clinical officer for SEND in the NHS focusing on improving educational outcomes for disabled children.

Glossary of terms and abbreviations used in the text

Ableism: Discrimination of, and social prejudice against, disabled people.

ACES: Adverse childhood experiences.

Adaptive planning: Requires knowledge of the strengths and needs of learners and pro-actively (rather than reactively) adapting the pedagogy.

Adaptive teaching: Involves adaptive planning prior to the lesson and adjusting practice during the lesson.

ADHD: Attention deficit hyperactivity disorder.

Affect: Emotion or desire as influencing behaviour.

Affective teaching: Involves introducing a session and creating a sense of belonging amongst students, tapping into their emotional wellbeing (like a check-in/warm-up starter but meaningful to these particular students).

AHP: Allied health professional.

AI: Artificial intelligence.

Alternative and augmentative communication (AAC): Using structured systems to support communication – may be a combination of objects, photos, symbols, communication books, sign language or high-tech aids, depending on an individual's needs.

Alternative provision (AP): Full-time education arranged by a local authority for children who cannot attend school for another reason (i.e. are out of school) or excluded pupils. AP must meet the needs of these students and enable them to achieve good educational attainment level.

Articulation: How speech sounds are physically formed in the mouth and vocal tract.

ASC: Autistic spectrum condition.

CAMHS: Child and adolescent mental health service.

CYP: Children and young people.

Developmental language disorder: A neurodevelopmental condition that affects language learning, including understanding and language use.

Discourse: Conversational skill marked by turn-taking, awareness and maintaining of conversational 'rules', and progressing a conversational exchange.

DLD: Developmental language disorder.

EAL: English as an additional language.

ECEC: Early childhood education and care.

ELKLAN: Training to equip staff with knowledge and strategies to enhance children's speech, language and communication skills.

Emergent multilingual (EM): Children continuing to develop their heritage language/s in addition to English (often referred to as having **EAL**).

EYP: Early years practitioner.

Executive functions: A set of mental skills that support our activation, focus, effort, emotional regulation and memory. It includes working memory, flexible thinking and self-control. Individuals experiencing difficulties with executive functions will experience challenges with, for example, organising, remembering information and concentrating.

Facilitated communication: Where another persona enables communication by, for example, supporting physically to reach a symbol where physical limitations exist. It is dependent on detailed understanding and correct interpretation of the communicator's actions and intent.

GCSE: General Certificate of Secondary Education is an academic qualification in a range of subjects taken in England, Wales and Northern Ireland.

Graduated approach: A four-stage cycle of special educational needs (SEN) support consisting of assess, plan, do and review cycles, initiated at Wave 2 or 3 (see **waves of intervention**).

Grammar: The whole system and structure of a language that determines how words are sequenced and adapted, usually taken as consisting of syntax and morphology.

HL: Heritage language. Learned by its speakers at home as children, which may be difficult to fully develop due to insufficient input from the surrounding social environment, meaning speakers grow up with a different dominant language in which they become more competent.

HLTA: Higher level teaching assistant.

Inclusion: Education that includes everyone, with non-disabled and disabled people learning together in mainstream schools, colleges and universities.

Initiation: The act of beginning an interaction, the power or opportunity to act before others do.

Interaction: Reciprocal action with another, responding to and having an effect on another.

Intonation: The rise and fall of the voice in speaking, which can infer different meanings.

KS: Key Stage (of national curriculum), e.g. KS1.

Language register: A variety of a language determined by degree of formality and choice of vocabulary, pronunciation and syntax, e.g. home dialect, slang, legal language.

Managed move: A voluntary agreement between two schools, a child and their parent/carer used to initiate a process which leads to the transfer of a child to another school permanently.

Metalinguistics: The ability to think and talk about language explicitly, including its components and the rules and structures that govern it.

Monolingualism: Being able to understand and speak in only one language (multilingualism being more prevalent).

Multilingualism: The ability to understand and speak in more than one languages which may be learned simultaneously or sequentially.

NAHT: National association of headteachers.

Neurodevelopmental: To do with the development of the brain and mental skills such as thinking, reasoning, making sense of emotions and social dynamics.

Neurodivergence: When someone's brain processes, learns, and/or behaves differently from what is considered 'typical', meaning that person has different strengths and challenges.

Neurodiversity: People experience and interact with the world around them in many different ways; there is no one 'right' way of thinking, learning and behaving, and differences are not viewed as deficits.

NHS: National Health Service.

Oracy: The ability to communicate effectively through talk in different contexts and for different purposes.

Pedagogy: The theory of teaching, and teaching approaches.

Phonology: How speech sounds are organised and contrasted within a language.

PISA: Programme for international student assessment.

Pragmatics: How language is used in context, such as how speakers communicate their intentions, how listeners infer meanings and how social factors influence language use.

Presupposition: Assumption of another's knowledge – accurate understanding of this is required to know how much detail to give/not give in order to maintain coherence and success in a conversation exchange.

Psycholinguistics: The top-down and bottom-up linguistic and psychological processes through which language is processed (decoded) and created (encoded).

Psychological: Affecting or arising in the mind – can be related to the mental and emotional state of a person.

Pupil referral unit (PRU): An alternative provision for pupils who are not able to attend mainstream school – often, but not exclusively, due to exclusion.

Quality first teaching (QFT): A style of teaching that focuses on high quality and inclusive teaching for every child in a classroom.

RCSLT: Royal College of Speech and Language Therapists.

SaLT: Speech and language therapy/speech and language therapist.

Scaffolding: A system of support that helps an individual learn new skills and concepts by providing tools and guidance or by breaking them into smaller chunks, which may be reduced once these have been mastered.

School exclusion: When a child is removed for either a temporary fixed term, or permanently, from a school for disciplinary reasons.

SEAL: Social and emotional aspects of learning.

SEL: Social and emotional learning.

Semantics: The meaning present in words/language.

SEMH: Social, emotional and mental health.

SEN(D): Special educational needs (and disability).

SEN(D)Co: The special educational needs (Disability) coordinator is responsible for leading the school or setting's provision for special educational needs (SEN) and coordinating the support offered to students with SEN.

SENDIASS: Special educational needs and disability information and advisory support service.

SLA: Service level agreement.

SLC: Speech, language and communication.

SLCN: Speech, language and communication needs.

SPD: Sensory processing disorder.

Speech sounds: The vocal sounds we use to make up the words of a language. Saying the right sounds in the right order is what allows us to successfully communicate with other people as all languages have their own set of sounds and rules about how these are combined (see **phonology**).

SpLD: Specific learning difficulty.

Stammering: Also known as stuttering. A speech condition characterised by repetition of sounds, syllables or words, stretching out sounds, or getting stuck or blocked when speaking.

TA: Teaching assistant.

Waves of intervention: Additional support for children with special educational needs delivered via three successive levels or 'waves':

> **Wave 1** is the expectation of 'quality first' teaching, supported by whole-school planning.
>
> **Wave 2** is more targeted support such as nurture groups, therapies, identified interventions and some 1:1 support.
>
> **Wave 3** usually involves an external specialist who advises on specialised support.

Created with reference to Our DEI Glossary (https://www.thebelongingeffect.co.uk/our-dei-glossary/) and in collaboration with Shannon Ludgate and Ellie Hill.

Introduction

Purpose

This book recognises, in line with Millard and Gaunt (2018:1) that *'speech and communication lie at the heart of classroom practice. It is the predominant way in which teachers provide instruction and support to their students and is central to how most students engage with the curriculum'*. This fact, however, has implications for teachers since approximately 1.9 million children in this country (1 in 5 pupils) are behind with talking and understanding of words and increasing delays in speech and language development are being recognised (Speech and Language UK, 2023). This means that student proficiency with speech, language and communication is not a given – a fact that in turn, has implications for how our CYP can access instruction, engage with the curriculum and so achieve.

We know that speech, language and communication (SLC) needs are the highest primary area of special education needs and are steadily rising (245,232 in January 2021, 262,416 in January 2022, 278,600 in June 2023, DfE 2023, 2024). Children are therefore entering nursery and school with lower baselines in speaking and listening skills (RCSLT, 2024). We also know communication and interaction skills involve all areas of life, being central to social and emotional wellbeing, and to learning, literacy and achievement. Increasing difficulties with these skills means there is a pressing need to act. However, practitioners in early years and in compulsory education phases require confidence, knowledge and skills to develop SLC skills in practice (Bercow, 2018; Gross, 2022).

Good teaching for pupils with SLC needs is good teaching for all. The initial teacher training (ITT) core content framework has been designed in the knowledge that the quality of teaching is the most important factor in improving outcomes for pupils – particularly pupils from disadvantaged backgrounds and those with additional needs (DfE, 2019). The White Paper (Gov.uk, 2022) and SEND Review (Gov.uk, 2023) therefore seek to improve provision through excellent teacher training and development and through a 'what works' evidence programme. However, The ITT Core Content *"deliberately does not detail approaches specific to particular additional needs – to reflect the importance of quality first teaching*" (p 5) and teachers identify gaps in their training and confidence supporting children and young people (CYP) with SLC needs (Dockrell and Howell, 2015; Dockrell et al. 2017).

This contrasts with Allen (2024) who suggests school leaders must acknowledge that prioritising the development of children's oracy skills is an urgent matter of social justice. This means it needs to be planned for and systematically taught which requires teacher professional development. There is therefore a need to equip practitioners with the knowledge and skills needed to embed pedagogical approaches at a universal level rather than just at targeted level and above.

This book seeks to develop teachers' knowledge of how to support SLC development and why these approaches work so they can support CYP to develop their SLC skills through the teaching and learning process and so enhance outcomes. The book aims to equip practitioners with knowledge, skills and resources to enhance their support of SLC skills; to demystify aspects of SLC through sharing of knowledge and theory; to build approaches that work upon this knowledge and to produce a text that bridges between education and speech and language therapy (SLT). We want to move away from comparing children to the 'norm' model, to person-centred care that foregrounds universal and targeted pedagogy. And we want you, the reader to see that supporting and developing SLC skills will enhance your pedagogy and support the work you do with these CYP on a day-to-day basis.

The first section of the book introduces foundational concepts. Chapter 1 explores the role SLC can play in the classroom and considers what an inclusive pedagogy might look like. Chapter 2 explores attention and listening abilities and how they underlie the development of SLC skills and are necessary for most learning and achievement. In Chapter 3, concept development and the contribution play makes to this is considered. Next, the dynamic relationship between emotional regulation in the classroom and why CYP experiencing SLC needs can be more prone to experiencing frustration are considered in Chapter 4. Chapter 5 centralises multilingualism, explaining that most of the world are multilingual and how language develops in children exposed to more than one language.

The second section of the book considers some specific SLC areas. Chapter 6 describes typical and atypical development of speech sounds and discusses links between speech sound development and CYP outcomes for learning, literacy, language and wellbeing. Chapter 7 focuses on the language we use within teaching, how we embed language teaching within the curriculum and how we can identify children who are finding understanding and use of language challenging. In Chapter 8, links between language and literacy are explained, including how conceptual knowledge (to which language labels/words are attached) is embedded in pedagogy and within a child's sociocultural learning environment, why speech and language therapists may have a role in some elements of literacy, and 'red flags' which might indicate that a CYP has difficulties with language that are impacting on their reading and writing. Next, communication intent and social interaction, how they develop and their import for pupil outcomes and wellbeing are explored in Chapter 9, before Chapter 10 examines the nature of stammering and its impact on CYP. The two remaining chapters in this section consider how social, emotional and mental health (SEMH) needs can be related to, often undiagnosed, SLC needs Chapter 11), and explore the relationship between SLC needs and school exclusion (Chapter 12).

The third and final section of the book outlines the importance of looking to the future and preparing CYP with SLC needs for adulthood, proposing measures that further education and higher education institutions can use (Chapter 13). It also considers how to create inclusive environments that maximise functional speech, language and communication practice (Chapter 14) and then goes on to explore interprofessional and collaborative working (Chapter 15).

How to use this book

We appreciate you are busy teachers who may simply be looking for answers.

- Each chapter stands alone so if you are coming to this book with a problem e.g. a child not focusing in class, you can dip into the chapter relevant to that area only.
- Each chapter provides knowledge and theory to develop your understanding and facilitate adaptation for your specific CYP. Information about how key skills and different aspects of speech, language and communication develop are provided to increase your awareness of when/how difficulties might appear and to help you to more easily recognise, assess and seek help for the CYP under your care.
- Critical questions are included to enable you to consider how you recognise and meet the area being considered e.g. emotional regulation.
- Perhaps most importantly, each chapter includes adaptive teaching strategies and resources, indicated in the text by the support icon:

You are encouraged to consider how these could work/be embedded in your specific setting, which may include identifying changes to be made to facilitate this.

To assist you to navigate and access the content, a glossary of terms, jointly created by educationalist and speech and language therapists is included. This is because terminology can seem like a whole other language. Terms used consistently throughout the book are therefore identified and reasons for these choices are explained as are any contentions surrounding them. This includes details of the abbreviations and acronyms used in the book.

Finally, we recognise there will be times when the assessment, advice and support of a speech and language therapist or other professionals will be necessary. These are indicated by the SoS icon:

accompanied by detail to look out for which may indicate a CYP is having significant difficulties that may be worth investigating further.

NB: We could not cover everything in detail but have kept the focus on the most important issues, knowledge and skills in what is meant to be an accessible resource that we really hope will become dog-eared with use.

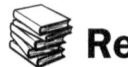 **References**

Allen, E (2024) Oracy: The urgent need for change and the role of schools as change agents. Available at: https://oracycambridge.org/schools-as-change-agents/ (accessed 7 January 2025).

Bercow (2018) Bercow: Ten Years On – An independent review of provision for children and young people with speech, language and communication needs in England. Available at http://www.bercow10yearson.com/ (accessed 7 January 2025).

DfE (2019) ITT Core Content Framework. Available at: ITT Core Content Framework (https://assets.publishing.service.gov.uk/media/6061eb9cd3bf7f5cde260984/ITT_core_content_framework_.pdf) (accessed 7 January 2025).

DfE (2023) Special educational needs in England: January 2023. Available at: Special educational needs in England: January 2023 – GOV.UK (https://www.gov.uk/government/statistics/special-educational-needs-in-england-january-2023) (accessed 7 January 2025).

DfE (2024) Special educational needs in England, June 2024. Available at: Special educational needs in England, Academic year 2023/24 – Explore education statistics - GOV.UK (https://explore-education-statistics.service.gov.uk/find-statistics.special-educational-needs-in-england) (accessed 7 January 2025).

Dockrell, J, and Howell, P (2015) Identifying the challenges and opportunities to meet the needs of children with speech, language, and communication difficulties. *British Journal of Special Education*, 42(4): 411–428.

Dockrell, J, Howell, P, Leung, D, and Fugard, A (2017) Children with speech language and communication needs in England: Challenges for practice. *Frontier Education*, 2(35): 1–14.

EEF (Educational Endowment Foundation) (2022) Special Educational Needs in Mainstream Schools—Recommendations (https://d2tic4wvo1iusb.cloudfront.net/production/eef-guidance-reports/send/EEF_Special_Educational_Needs_in_Mainstream_Schools_Recommendations_Poster.pdf?v=1727858166) (accessed 7 January 2025).

Gov.uk (2022) Opportunity for all Strong schools with great teachers for your child. Available at: Opportunity for all – Strong schools with great teachers for your child (https://assets.publishing.service.gov.uk/media/62416cb5d3bf7f32add7819f/Opportunity_for_all_strong_schools_with_great_teachers_for_your_child__print_version_.pdf) (accessed 7 January 2025).

Gov.uk (2023) SEND Review: right support, right place, right time. Available at: SEND Review Summary document (https://assets.publishing.service.gov.uk/media/62445269d3bf7f32afeba006/SEND_Review_Right_support_right_place_right_time_summary.pdf) (accessed 7 January 2025).

Gross, J (2022) *Reaching the Unseen Children: Practical Strategies for Closing Stubborn Attainment Gaps in Disadvantaged Groups*. Abingdon, UK: Routledge.

Miller, W, and Gaunt, A (2018) Speaking up: The importance of oracy in teaching and learning. *Impact* 3: 12–15. Available at: Speaking up: The importance of oracy in teaching and learning (https://my.chartered.college/impact_article/speaking-up-the-importance-of-oracy-in-teaching-and-learning/) (accessed 7 January 2025).

Millard, W and Gaunt, A (2018) Speaking up: The importance of oracy in teaching and learning (https://my.chartered.college/impact_article/speaking-up-the-importance-of-oracy-in-teaching-and-learning/) (accessed 7 January 2024).

RCSLT (2024) We are the Village: Speech, Language and Communication in the Early Years. Early-years_We-are-the-Village-report_NI_April-2024.pdf (https://www.rcslt.org/wp-content/uploads/2024/04/Early-years_We-are-the-Village-report_NI_April-2024.pdf).

Speech and Language UK (2023) Listening to unheard children: a shocking rise in speech and language challenges. Available at: Listening-to-unheard-children-report-FINAL.pdf (https://speechandlanguage.org.uk/wp-content/uploads/2024/03/Listening-to-unheard-children-report-FINAL.pdf) (accessed 7 January 2025).

SECTION I FUNDAMENTALS

1 Inclusive pedagogy for supporting speech, language and communication

Stephanie Brewster

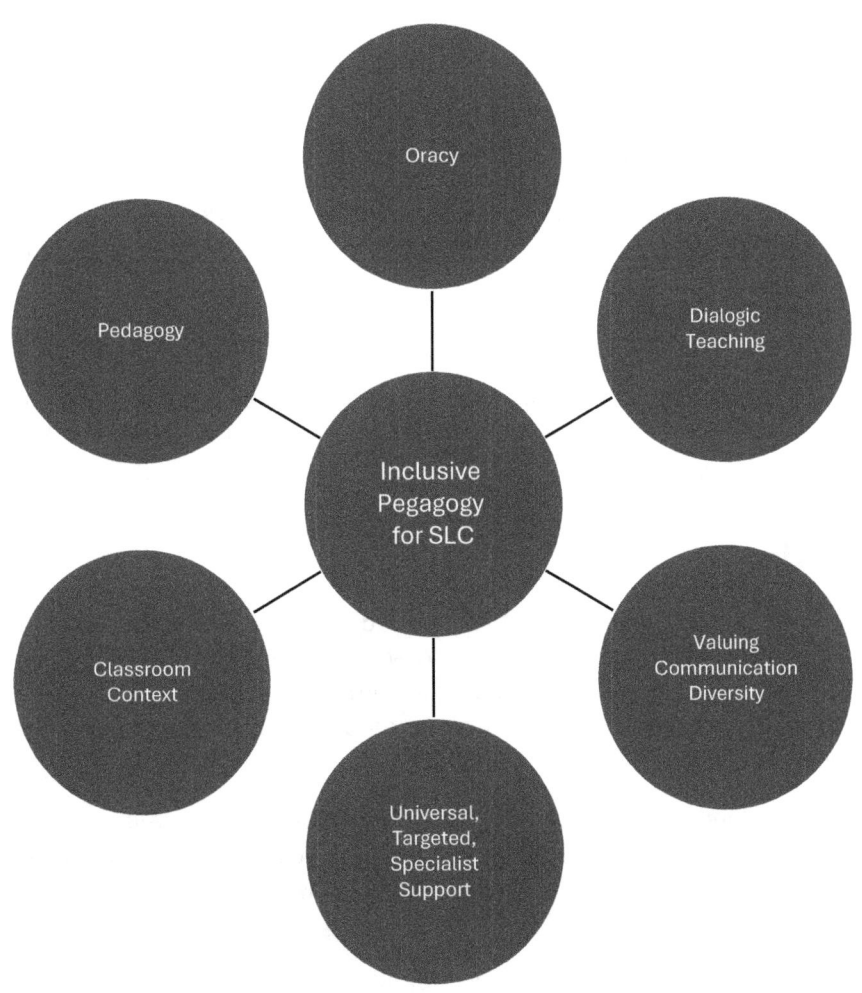

DOI: 10.4324/9781041054986-3

CHAPTER OBJECTIVES

The chapter:

- Explores the concept of pedagogy arguing that speech, language and communication (SLC) is central to inclusive pedagogy;
- Considers universal approaches for promoting talk-based pedagogy, with particular reference to oracy and dialogic teaching;
- Examines the implications for pupils with SLC needs requiring targeted and specialist interventions;
- Reflects on the diversity and variation in communication presented by pupils;
- Suggests a range of practitioner resources.

CRITICAL QUESTION

Talk makes a unique and powerful contribution to children's development, thinking and learning, and [...] it must therefore have a central place in their education.

(Alexander, 2020, p. 19)

- To what extent does your practice as an education professional reflect the intentional use of speaking, listening and communication in the classroom?

Introduction

As a reader of this book, you are probably already aware of the importance of speech, language and communication (SLC) for children and young people, and Chapter 1 will help you to more explicitly evidence and articulate this position. It is a position that is widely shared by others, and variously framed as a matter of democracy, social justice, social mobility, equity and inclusion. Education is central to these endeavours.

According to the landmark Bercow report (DCSF, 2008, p. 17), '*Almost all aspects of school life are language based*'. Yet, despite concerns about increasing speech, language and communication needs (SLCN) in recent years, many education professionals are still ill-equipped to address them.

This chapter argues that explicitly and systematically teaching spoken language skills (Allen, 2024) both supports the development of those skills and enhances learning across the entire curriculum for all pupils, at all stages. SLC should play a central role in any universally provided pedagogy; but there are also risks for those pupils needing more targeted or specialist provision. Below, we consider these implications, drawing on the notion of pedagogy to support our discussion.

Pedagogy

While not a concept that is widely used or fully understood in English education, 'pedagogy' provides a useful perspective. Rozsahegyi and Lambert (2016) convey the breadth of the concept: on one hand it encompasses the theory, attitudes, values, principles, philosophy and ethics of education; and on the other, the social practice, teaching activities and strategies employed within education. It goes beyond concern for formal learning outcomes, to a holistic *'commitment to children's overall development'* (Rozsahegyi and Lambert 2016, p. 41). Pedagogical principles are common to all ages/phases, while practical strategies are implemented differently in different contexts.

Rozsahegyi and Lambert (2016) raise the question: *'to what extent does the nature of pedagogy apply in the same way to all learners?'* (p. 45). An inclusive pedagogy is universal and based on what all learners have in common. If high quality, Rozsahegyi and Lambert argue, then logically this results in fewer pupils being labelled and categorised as having needs that are 'special' or 'additional' to those of others.

It is rarely explicitly identified that the conceptualisations of pedagogy indicated above imply the centrality of social interaction within teaching and learning activities: pedagogy is inherently a social framework. Oracy and dialogic teaching (discussed below) are manifestations of the foregrounding of communication in an educational context. However, such broad pedagogical approaches which emphasise SLC are still underdeveloped when it comes to addressing individual needs in this area; and conversely, literature on SLCN often makes little or no reference to pedagogy.

Pedagogy also covers systemic issues of the management of education and curriculum, as reflected in policy. It has long been the case in English educational policy that 'speaking and listening' are primarily seen as a foundation for subsequent literacy (which of course they are), rather than as a worthy end in their own right. As Alexander points out (2020), raising the profile of speaking and listening enhances rather than detracts from the teaching of literacy, despite the common fears of policymakers that the opposite is true. Unfortunately, *'speaking and listening is no longer a discrete curriculum area with its own defined age progression'* (Gross, 2017, p. 3) in the National Curriculum, which provides insufficient guidance to teachers about how to *'meet its ambition for spoken language'* (Oracy Education Commission, 2024, p. 22).

Despite this, skilled teachers maximise classroom interaction, using every opportunity to model the use of rich language, and to develop this in their pupils. Such teachers see themselves as facilitators of pupils' active and collaborative construction of knowledge and understanding through classroom interaction. This view of learning is based on the social constructivist theory of learning. According to this, cognitive development is not only a biological process but also a social one, in which the learner constructs meaning through interaction with others, usually through spoken language (Alexander, 2020). Interaction is essential for acquiring and understanding knowledge, and also for the development of identity and a sense of self. Coultas (2015, p. 73) refers to Vygotsky's view that learning is inherently social and that *'talk is essential in organising our thoughts and extending our thinking'*. This perspective is often evident in the classroom in the form of scaffolding, through which support offered within interaction is carefully tailored to the learner's current level of performance and gradually reduced, allowing the learner to develop independent mastery.

The classroom context

The theoretical perspectives outlined above indicate how communication is not only a legitimate curriculum area but is also a fundamental underpinning of learning more broadly. This is true of all phases of education, despite the tendency to place SLC as lower priority in later phases (Oracy All Party Parliamentary Group, 2021).

Supporting SLC development for the youngest children is, rightly, prioritised in the EYFS and Key Stage 1, and early years' practitioners appreciate the importance of engaging with the child's home learning environment. This is recognised as particularly important in areas of social disadvantage (Gascoigne and Gross, 2017) where, research suggests, half of children starting school will have SLCN: a pattern which persists into secondary level. However, we should caution against assuming that the link between social disadvantage and SLCN is necessarily one of causation: as Gross (2017) says, coming from a well-off family does not always result in a richer home communication environment and therefore greater language skills.

Beyond the early years, pupils still need a sustained focus on SLC. In the secondary level, for example, the language demands of schooling increase significantly: ideas and language become more abstract, there is increased use of inference and figurative language, greater grammatical complexity, and additional technical vocabulary associated with curriculum subjects (See Chapter 12).

The current educational response to the provision of support often follows a 'waves of intervention' model:

- **Wave 1**: provision of 'Quality First Teaching', through inclusive universal pedagogy, evident in whole school approaches which meet most pupils' needs;
- **Wave 2**: targeted additional support for a smaller proportion of pupils;
- **Wave 3**: specialist assessment and interventions for a small minority of pupils whose needs may be regarded as a clinical (within-child) or biologically based disorder.

SLCN is a useful catch-all term that encompasses all SLC needs, whether associated with a specific condition (e.g. Developmental Language Disorder), part of a wider profile of SEND, or delayed development of communication skills (Gascoigne and Gross, 2017).

There is no clear distinction between a 'special educational needs' (SEN) issue and developmental variation, and social factors affecting development of SLC always need consideration.

Given the high prevalence of SLCN of some sort (see Introduction p. 1), there is a strong case for a pedagogy that accounts for such needs from the outset. Indeed, the better the universal provision, the lower the need for targeted or specialist support. Oracy is the current conceptualisation of such universal pedagogies which place SLC at the centre.

Oracy

The increasing profile of oracy reflects a deepening appreciation of the importance of *'Articulating ideas, developing understanding and engaging with others through speaking, listening and communication'* (Oracy Education Commission, 2024, p. 8). Oracy education is the intentional cultivation of these abilities, through

- 'learning *to* talk' (a developmental perspective through which spoken language skills are a curricular goal in their own right) and
- 'learning *through* talk' (i.e. talk as pedagogy or process).

(Oracy Benchmarks, Voice21, 2019, p. 3)

The Oracy benchmarks (Voice21, 2020) aim to address the lack of guidance and support for teachers regarding such approaches. A key point of reference is the Oracy Framework (2021) which identifies four strands:

- physical (voice, body language)
- linguistic (including vocabulary and rhetorical techniques)
- cognitive (including content and structure)
- social and emotional (such as working with others, confidence, listening)

However, the current interpretation of 'oracy' has received considerable criticism (see Chapter 9). The framework emphasises the external or observable features of effective communication. But superficial matters such as clarity of speech are less significant than a pupil's underlying capacity to listen, pay attention, interact, understand language and to express themselves through meaningful vocabulary and language structure.

Recently, attempts have been made to rebalance the underplay of listening in oracy; for example, the Oracy Education Commission's 2024 report replaces '*talk*' with '*talk, listen and communicate*'. This phrase places equal emphasis on listening and speaking, and enables the recognition of other forms of communication such as sign language or augmentative or alternative communication. The report also defines a third component of oracy:

- learning *about* talk, listening and communication: '*building knowledge and understanding of speaking, listening and communication in its many contexts*' (p. 14).

Only the 'learning *through* talk' strand of oracy entails the social constructivist theory of learning discussed earlier this strand focuses on pupil and teacher thinking together and engaging in dialogue.

Dialogic teaching

Teachers typically do most of the talking in class, controlling what is said, and who says it (Alexander, 2020). Teacher talk often risks closing down classroom interaction, through questions which are closed and designed to elicit a 'correct' answer. This does not support the kind of sustained interaction which exploits the developmental and pedagogical power of classroom talk.

Dialogic teaching is a universal pedagogical approach that addresses these limitations. Embedded within the wider concept of dialogic inquiry, whereby pupils and teachers co-construct knowledge, dialogue (comprising both teacher-pupil and pupil-pupil speaking and listening) holds significant potential for promoting pupils' active participation in learning (Pollard, 2023).

There is now a robust body of research evidence of the effectiveness of dialogic teaching in terms of additional progress in standardised tests in English, maths and science. When talk is '*well-structured and cognitively demanding*', there is a direct positive impact on student engagement and learning (Alexander, 2020, p. 19). Pollard (2023) draws particular attention to the importance of carefully managed collaborative group work within a dialogic approach, along with teachers' use of sophisticated questioning techniques. Indeed, dialogic teaching requires teachers to have a broad repertoire of interactional strategies (Alexander, 2020) which aim to provide '*authentic opportunities for reasoned discussion in class*' (Gross, 2017, p. 2). Such discussions fulfil a number of functions, including thinking, learning, communicating, teaching and assessing (Alexander, 2020). Classroom dialogue also facilitates the identification of needs and assessment of progress, which is particularly important for pupils with SLCN; however, whether such pedagogic processes can be fully inclusive, is considered in the next section.

How inclusive are 'talk'-based pedagogies?

It is important to ask who benefits most from universal pedagogies that place interaction at their core. While the case for a much stronger emphasis on talk in educational policy and practice is strong and persuasive, there are risks of disadvantaging many specific groups of pupils, those with SLCN among them.

It could be argued that the whole concept of 'oracy' implies an exclusive focus on speaking/listening modalities of communication (or at least giving primacy to these), to the exclusion of other modes of interaction such as sign language, or asynchronous interaction styles preferred by some neurodivergent children (Reeves and Wright, 2024).

Furthermore, Cushing (2024) has been highly critical of the common claims that oracy can be used to '*close disadvantage gaps*' and '*promote social equity*' (Voice21, no date). Cushing argues that oracy is *not* effective in tackling the social disadvantage experienced by marginalised (particularly working-class and racialised) children and young people, since the roots of inequality are structural and cannot be remediated by '*making tweaks to their language*' (p. 1). The oracy agenda all too often entails assumptions of the '*deficient language practices of marginalised communities*' (Cushing, 2024, p. 3), which differ from (and are thereby seen as inferior to) white middle-class language patterns. But as Cushing points out, '*working-class children have vast stylistic repertoires which they consciously and dexterously draw from*' (p. 7), but which are devalued in the classroom.

The expectations of the Oracy Framework (2021) are problematic for other groups of pupils too. For example, the requirement for students to speak in class may provoke anxiety for a shy child, one for whom it takes time to put thoughts into words, or who fears 'saying the wrong thing', and those naturally preferring to think and listen rather than speak. These pupils may be judged as un-engaged or unwilling to participate (Alexander, 2020), and may even experience unintended harm through just such a '*non-inclusive approach to oracy education*' (Reeves and Wright, 2024, p. 15). And yet exempting them from oracy activity could entrench their disadvantage even further.

Valuing communicative diversity

In response to the above concerns, there is a growing recognition of pupils' communicative diversity and the need to ensure that classroom interaction does not constrain or diminish pupils' natural communication styles and preferences. This, however, is not reflected in current English educational policy. The National Curriculum emphasises use of traditional models of presentational talk and Standard English. This potentially devalues diverse linguistic backgrounds, atypical modes of communication and also other modes of classroom interaction such as exploratory talk – in which pupils collaborate towards a shared purpose (Gaunt and Stott, 2019) – and informal peer-to-peer interactional styles. If language is only viewed as a tool of instruction, didactic closed questioning will dominate, and non-Standard English will be corrected, thereby sending a clear message about the unacceptability of non-standard varieties of language (Coultas, 2015 p. 79).

Snell (2024) advocates viewing variation in (spoken) language as a resource, such that choices can be made appropriate to the specific context of the interaction. Learning *about* talk, listening and communication (Oracy Education Commission, 2024), and giving pupils '*a range of opportunities to use different talk repertoires*' (Coultas, 2015, p. 72), empowers pupils to make conscious choices about language use and understand the choices of others, including the implications of race, class and other speaker characteristics.

> ⓘ **CRITICAL QUESTIONS**
>
> - How can teachers listen deeply to, recognise the validity of and celebrate diverse linguistic repertoires and communication practices?
> - How can you simultaneously support the development of effective communication skills and learning of Standard English?

Identification and assessment for SLCN

So far, we have considered how universal approaches which maximise classroom interaction can support all pupils' SLC development, and their learning more broadly. However, with on average two children in every class of 30 (Gascoigne and Gross, 2017) likely to have Developmental Language Disorder requiring targeted and/or specialist intervention, education practitioners must be able to quickly identify when such intervention is needed.

There is much evidence of under-identification and yet screening is still not comprehensively conducted, despite the many readily available screening tools for children of all ages. The Oracy Education Commission (2024) points out that half of teachers do not feel they have had sufficient training to adequately support their pupils' speech and language development; hence, there is still a major need for developing the education workforce. This is particularly the case in later phases of education where the focus is increasingly on preparing learners for their transition into employment (see Chapter 12). However, while the vast majority of employers need their workforce to have strong spoken communication skills above all else, only a minority of teachers recognise this.

Talk can also be a powerful assessment tool in terms of both assessment of and for learning. As Alexander (2020, p. 1) puts it, dialogic teaching is helpful because '*by encouraging students to share their thinking, it enables teachers to diagnose needs, devise learning tasks, enhance understanding, assess progress*'. This is all the more important, though harder to achieve, where pupils' SLC needs create challenges for gathering evidence of their progress and achievement.

Targeted and specialist intervention

Earlier it was pointed out that some pupils may not be able to meet conventional expectations of oracy. This may be even more likely for those with a communication impairment. Eye contact may be challenging for autistic pupils; facial expression and body language for those with motor conditions may not look how we would expect them to. Any focus on confidence, fluency, pace of speech and self-assurance will clearly disadvantage pupils with Developmental Language Disorder, pupils who stammer (see Chapter 10), and users of alternative methods of communication. The same can be said for pupils with non-standard dialects and those who use English as an additional language (EAL) and are new to English. Pupils with EAL make up an increasing proportion of the UK school population (see Chapter 5); they are likely to need additional support in acquiring English, and some will also have SLCN and/or SEN.

An inclusive learning environment and universal educational practices promoting SLC – however, inclusively these are interpreted – will still not be enough for the smaller numbers of pupils for whom targeted or specialist intervention is needed. When identifying pupils for targeted intervention, care must be taken not to assume an SLC deficit based on their home background or marginalised status (see above).

Speech and language disorders secondary to a primary impairment, such as hearing loss/impairment, physical impairment or intellectual/learning disability, or Developmental Language Disorder, all indicate a likely need for more specialist, often individual intervention. Since it cannot be assumed that all such pupils will already be known to external specialist services, it is essential that teachers know when and how to make referrals. However, the involvement of a speech and language therapist does not mean the teacher hands over responsibility for the pupil's acquisition and generalisation of new SLC skills, but rather that they work collaboratively towards the practical implementation of mutually agreed strategies within the school environment.

Applicable to both targeted work under the guidance of the teacher, and to delivery of specialist interventions indicated by an SLT, Radford (2017) highlights the role of the teaching assistant. The TA will often be a key interaction partner for pupils with SLCN, engaging in scaffolding which provides a linguistic model for the pupil. Doing so in such a way that does not foster dependency but promotes learning of and through language requires considerable skill; this has significant implications for the professional development of the TA and others who support children with SLCN (see below for suggested resources).

CASE STUDY

Lucy, class teacher and inclusion lead in an inner city mainstream junior school, Key Stage 2 (7–11 year-old pupils)

Recent years have seen progress in supporting very young children's communication and language development – one of the three prime areas of the Early Years Foundation Stage statutory framework. But there is no assessment of speech and language after the age of five, and speaking and listening has been removed from the primary National Curriculum. So, I feel more needs to be done to support learners over the age of five with SLCN, particularly in areas of social deprivation, like where my school is situated. This is key to effective inclusion, which should enable the innate motivation of pupils with communication needs to interact and flourish within their educational settings.

Conducting various learning walks within my setting, I found that some colleagues needed greater knowledge of SLCN to help them identify individualised learning targets. But I also think that purely individualised approaches do not solve the difficulties, but instead reinforce that there is a significant problem (Florian, 2017). I also found that some colleagues struggled to encourage talk or peer interaction for the purpose of actively inspiring curiosity and exploration. Much of the classroom talk involved heavy use of teacher instruction, which could cause some pupils to disengage and feel overwhelmed.

Our setting recognised the importance of timely access to specialist provision for pupils with the most complex SLCN, but our area '*has historically been one of the poorest funded areas [for speech and language therapy services] despite significant levels of deprivation across the region'* (Rudd, 2023). We therefore needed to consider ways of developing our own expertise.

- The teaching team decided to focus on the use of language in the classroom to create the element of surprise, to encourage pupils with SLCN to communicate with others and immerse themselves in an exciting learning environment. This worked well for a pupil with receptive and expressive language difficulties, who was excited to experience a surprise role play area linked to *Goldilocks and the Three Bears* which the class had been studying in their English lessons. This enabled them to feel and communicate the surprise felt by the characters in the story, and to connect their own experience with the characters.
- At a whole school level, part of the notional SEN budget was used to fund professional development opportunities around SLCN. With a colleague, I also conducted training in specific interventions, such as Memory Magic (Booth, 2009) which was highly effective in supporting many children with retaining key language and stimulating social interaction.
- Community-wide, a new hub offered parents ESOL (English for speakers of other languages) classes and parent workshops. We observed that targeting specific parents with early support and language-enhancement opportunities, often positively influenced children's progress and parental support for specialist intervention.

⑦ Critical questions

- How can you create 'real' (purposeful, meaningful and personal) communication opportunities in the classroom?
- Each pupil must feel they are included and valued before they freely interact with others. How can you extend the quality of communication-enhancing provision for all your pupils?

References

Booth, J (2009) Memory Magic. Elklan. Available at: www.elklan.co.uk/Shop/Memory_Magic (accessed 21 December 2024).

Florian, L (2017) The concept of inclusive pedagogy. In: Hallett, F and Hallett, G (eds) *Transforming the Role of the SENCO*. London: OU Press.

Rudd, G (2023) *'Unheard children' must not be ignored following worrying report into speech and language issues*. Birmingham City University. Available at: www.bcu.ac.uk/news-events/news/unheard-children-must-not-be-ignored-following-worrying-report-into-speech-and-language-issues (accessed 21 December 2024).

INFORMATION AND RESOURCES FOR EDUCATORS

There is so much material now freely available it can be hard to know where to start; creating a communication-supportive classroom environment is a good initial goal. (see also Chapter 14). Gross (2017) suggests many practical whole-class strategies, organised around the following themes:

- A place to talk – creating a rich language-learning environment; this could be through creating 'hot-spots' which stimulate interaction e.g. through role play areas equipped with physical resources which prompt collaboration.
- A reason to talk – providing opportunities for authentic interaction through, for example, creating surprise, pupils asking questions and giving instructions, collaborating, debating, drama and role play.
- Actively teaching aspects of communication such as vocabulary, listening skills and comprehension.

A wealth of further resources can be found online, for example:

- Speech Language and Communication Framework www.slcframework.org.uk/

A professional development tool and searchable resource database.

- Education Endowment Foundation https://educationendowmentfoundation.org.uk

Provides a searchable database of evidence-based resources e.g. Oral Language Interventions.

- AFASIC www.afasic.org.uk/

A source of support and information for families of children with SLCN.

- Speech and Language UK https://speechandlanguage.org.uk/

You may be most interested in the Educators and Professionals Resource Library, and the What Works database of evidenced interventions.

- ICAN www.icancharity.org.uk/

Provides an independent assessment service, training for the children's workforce, and resources.

- Nasen https://nasen.org.uk/

Provides information, training and resources to members, on all aspects of SEND, including SLCN.

- Voice21 https://voice21.org/

The UK's oracy education charity, which works with member schools.

- Oracy Cambridge https://oracycambridge.org/

Promotes oracy through its publications, training and consultancy activities.

- Mesh Guides www.new.meshguides.org/

Provides A-Z summaries of research-based specialist knowledge for educators, for example, Classroom Dialogue and Learning.

CHAPTER SUMMARY

- This chapter explored the role SLC can play in the classroom, and considered what an inclusive pedagogy might look like. A language-rich environment is essential to universal educational provision, for all ages, a focus which is captured by the notion of 'oracy'.

- Learning *to* talk, listen and communicate is a curricular goal in its own right. Equally important is the pedagogical process of learning *through* talking, listening and communicating – using dialogic teaching across the entire curriculum.

- However, many groups of children, especially those with SLCN, are at risk of being disadvantaged by prevailing conceptualisations of oracy. Although the foregrounding of talk in the classroom can help teachers to identify and support such pupils, there are significant numbers not being spotted soon enough. Targeted and specialist provision are important if the SLC needs of all pupils are to be met.

- The role of communication in the classroom is under threat; without sufficient policy and inspection emphasis, teachers are not empowered to implement pedagogies which maximise the power of interaction in the classroom. There is a need for further research, guidance and training for teachers to implement pedagogies that are inclusive for all pupils including those with SLCN.

Further reading

Hayden, S and Jordan, E (2024) *Language for Learning in the Primary School: A Practical Guide for Supporting Pupils with Speech, Language and Communication Needs Across the Curriculum*. 3rd ed. Oxford: Routledge.

- A very practical text containing many useful resources, accompanied by online materials.

Knight, R (2020) *Classroom Talk: Evidence-based Teaching for Enquiring Teachers*. St Albans: Critical Publishing.
- Covering both theory and practice, this text examines the evidence relating to classroom talk.

Law, J (2019) The changing perception of communication needs: A litmus test for the Warnock Legacy. *Frontiers in Education*, 4:42, 1–9.
- This article considers how the term SLCN has played out across health and education services.

 References

Alexander, R (2020) *A Dialogic Teaching Companion*. Abingdon: Routledge.

Allen, E (2024) Oracy: The urgent need for change and the role of schools as change agents. Oracy Cambridge. Available at: https://oracycambridge.org/schools-as-change-agents/ (accessed 6 March 2025).

Coultas, V (2015) Revisiting debates on oracy: Classroom talk -moving towards a democratic pedagogy? *Changing English; Studies in Culture and Education*, 22(1): 72–86.

Cushing, I (2024) Social in/justice and the deficit foundations of oracy. *Oxford Review of Education*. Available at: Full article: Social in/justice and the deficit foundations of oracy (https://www.tandfonline.com/doi/full/10.1080/03054985.2024.2311134) (accessed 6 March 2025).

DCSF (2008) *The Bercow Report: A Review of Services for Children and Young People (0–19) with Speech, Language and Communication Needs*. Available at: https://dera.ioe.ac.uk/id/eprint/8405/7/7771-dcsf-bercow_Redacted.pdf (accessed 6 March 2025).

Gascoigne, M and Gross, J (2017) *Talking About a Generation; current policy, evidence and practice for speech, language and communication*. ICAN/The Communication Trust. Available at: www.bettercommunication.org.uk/downloads/ (accessed 6 March 2025).

Gaunt, A and Stott, A (2019) *Transform Teaching and Learning Through Talk: The Oracy Imperative*. Lanham: Rowman & Littlefield Publishers.

Gross, J (2017) *Time to Talk: Implementing Outstanding Practice in Speech, Language and Communication*. 2nd ed. London: Routledge.

Oracy All-Party Parliamentary Group Inquiry (2021) *Speak for Change*. Available at: https://voice21.org/wp-content/uploads/2024/01/Oracy_APPG_FinalReport_28_04-4.pdf (accessed 6 March 2025).

Oracy Education Commission (2024) *We Need to Talk; The report of the Commission on the Future of Oracy Education in England*. Available at https://oracyeducationcommission.co.uk/oec-report/ (accessed 6 March 2025).

Pollard, A (2023) *Reflective Teaching in Secondary Schools*. 6th ed. London: Bloomsbury

Radford, J A (2017) Helping language learning in inclusive classrooms. In Bar-On, A and Ravit, D, (eds) *Handbook of Communication Disorders: Theoretical, Empirical and Applied Linguistics Perspectives*. Berlin/Munich/Boston: De Gruyter.

Reeves, L and Wright, C (2024) *How Can Oracy Be Inclusive of Children and Young People with Communication Needs and Differences?* Speaking Volumes, London: The Oracy Education Commission. Available at: https://oracyeducationcommission.co.uk/wp-content/uploads/2024/09/Speaking-Volumes-OEC-v6b.pdf (accessed 6 March 2025).

Rozsahegyi, T and Lambert, M (2016) Pedagogy for inclusion? In Brown, Z (ed) *Inclusive Education*. Abingdon, UK: Routledge.

Snell, J (2024) *What Do Teachers Need to Learn About Oracy?* Speaking Volumes, London: The Oracy Education Commission. Available at: https://oracyeducationcommission.co.uk/wp-content/uploads/2024/09/Speaking-Volumes-OEC-v6b.pdf (accessed 6 March 2025).

Voice 21 (2020) The Oracy Benchmarks. Available at: https://voice21.org/wp-content/uploads/2020/06/Benchmarks-report-FINAL.pdf (accessed 6 March 2025).

Voice 21 and Oracy Cambridge (2021) The Oracy Framework. Available at: https://membership-hub.voice21.org/the-oracy-framework (accessed 6 March 2025).

2 Attention and listening

Hazel Richards

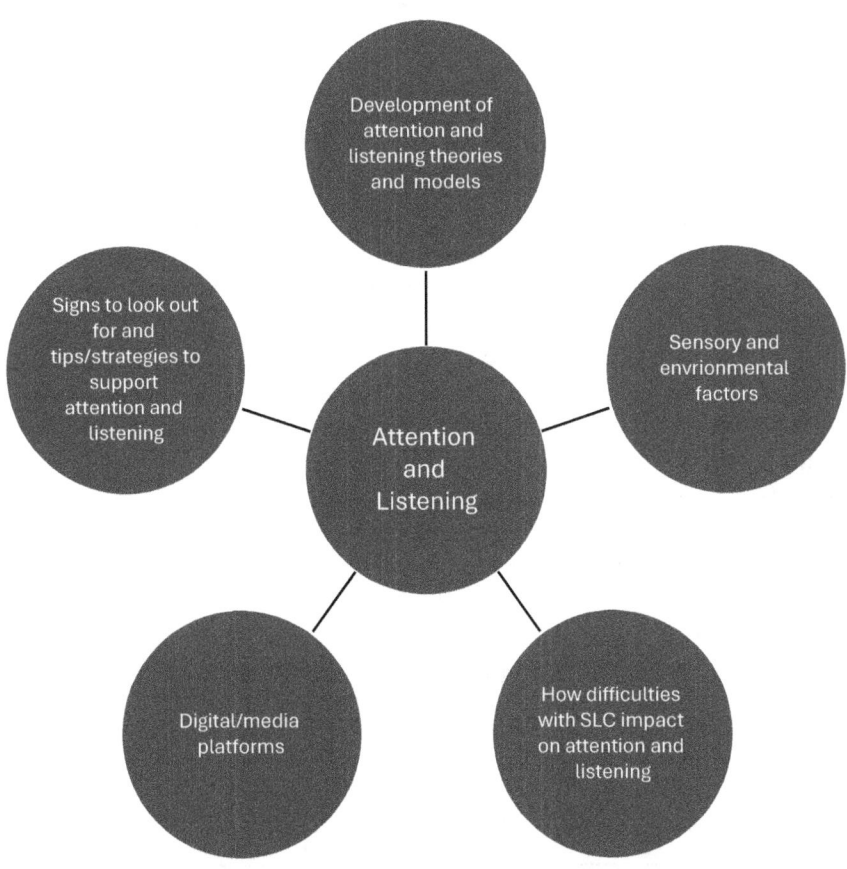

🎯 CHAPTER OBJECTIVES

This chapter explores the centrality of attention and listening for speech, language and communication (SLC) skills. The chapter:

- explores theories and models of attention and listening development;
- considers physical hearing, sensory and environmental factors;
- identifies how SLC skills can also impact attention and listening;
- considers conditions where attention and listening challenges are more likely to be present;
- ponders challenges created by digital media/platform multitasking; and
- details signs to look out for and provides tips and strategies to support different attention and listening levels.

Introduction

Mental processes, including attention and listening (as distinct from hearing) underlie speech, language and communication (SLC) skills. How we attend and listen, and how others attend and listen to us, directly impacts how our SLC skills develop, and our access to teaching and learning. This is because all teaching and learning requires attention and listening, with most delivery and assessment being language based. Targeting attention and listening skills through universal pedagogical strategies and reasonable adjustments incorporated into routine practice will therefore enhance the academic, social and life chances of all children and young people (CYP), not just those at risk of/with identified SLC needs.

🏁 STARTING POINTS

- How do you attend and listen to the children and young people you work with?
- How does this help you tune in and respond to them?
- How in turn, do they attend and listen to you?
- What import does this have for your teaching and their learning?

Attention

Attention is the ability to focus on specific information in the environment and involves prioritising what is important or interesting to you whilst disregarding other stimuli present. Attention helps us determine which elements in our environment we need to focus on and has been divided into:

- bottom-up processing: a *passive* attention driven by external stimuli and levels of alertness;
- top-down processing: requires conscious activation and effort, and is more *active*, that is, linked to goals and motivation.

Mirsky (1991) separated attention into four main components:

1. focusing attention;
2. sustaining it over time;
3. shifting attention from one thing to another;
4. mentally registering the information attended to through the process of encoding.

These processes take conscious effort and require attention control, which develops through childhood. Cooper et al. (1978) identified six stages of attention development (see Table 2.1):

Table 2.1 Cooper, Moodley and Reynell's (1978) six levels of attention development

Attention Development Level	Description	Strategies to Support
1. Fleeting attention	The individual is easily distracted and their attention flits between people and objects.	– Follow the CYP's lead/get into their world to build rapport. – Keep instructions simple and task related by using keywords only. – Model by showing the CYP what to do. – Use prompts to gain attention such as gestures, touching the CYP's arm or guiding them (as minimal guidance when/if appropriate). – Use objects/activities that are engaging and allow for many repetitions.
2. Rigid attention	The individual can concentrate on a task of their choosing but may not respond to their name being called (so may come across as rude) and finds it hard to refocus following interruption.	– Observe their activity, extending it where possible by demonstrating possibilities. – Encourage attention to sounds, for example, singing, musical instruments, activities involving different sounds. – Help the CYP refocus after a distraction, e.g. by calling their name, settling the class, etc.

(Continued)

Table 2.1 (Continued)

Attention Development Level	Description	Strategies to Support
3. Single-channelled attention	The individual can attend to an activity suggested/presented by another. They can follow simple instructions but cannot do this whilst simultaneously completing a task. This means you need to gain their attention before giving them an instruction as they can only focus on one thing at a time.	– Gain attention before giving short instructions. – Turn-taking and copying games can help develop focus. – Leave words out of well-known songs, stories or instructions to encourage attention and responses.
4. Focused attention	Although the individual can only concentrate on one thing at time, they can now shift their attention to an alternative activity without support. You may still need to call out their name to gain their initial attention but they can respond more quickly.	– Provide a carousel of activities, positioning staff to support and extend attention before the CYP moves to the next activity. – Provide novel problem-solving activities that introduce different stages in a task to sustain attention for longer.
5. Two-channelled attention	The individual is able to listen to instructions while completing another activity at the same time.	– Add additional instructions/suggestions as an activity progresses and support CYP to respond to/integrate these into the task. Provide visual formats of these to augment and support the spoken word.
6. Integrated attention	The individual can attend to activities without frequent reminding to stay on task and is able to attend to people and activities in numerous environments, juggling multiple stimuli successfully.	– Vary the people and contexts tasks are completed with/in to extend CYP's ability to integrate multiple components and still stay on/return to task. – Relate the learning content to real-life/relatable examples.

Whilst the levels in Table 2.1 are useful, other factors also contribute to attentional control. For example, CYP who have experienced trauma may shift to a heightened state of alertness when a threat is perceived, affecting how and what they attend to. We also know attention capacity is limited and varies according to motivation for, and perceived difficulty of the task being attended to. Memory and executive function skills are also involved.

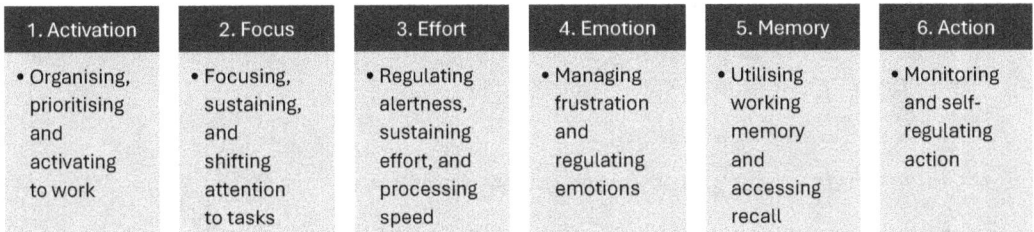

Figure 2.1 The six clusters of Brown's executive function model (Adapted from Brown, 2006, p. 39)

Memory is entwined with attention and essential for learning, problem-solving and speech, language and communication. Working memory allows us to temporarily hold and manipulate a finite amount of information for immediate mental use. Whereas short-term memory refers to temporary storage of information, working memory enables information to be processed, contributing to the representations we lay down in our long-term memory. How and what we attend to directly influences the information we receive and process, and therefore, how we make sense of this information and store it (Chapter 3, page 41-42). Different conceptualisations of executive function, the brain's cognitive management system, exist. Brown's model (2006) identifies six clusters of cognitive functions that work together in various ways:

Each of the cognitive functions (Figure 2.1) interact and have an influence on attention, hence why it is important to consider motivation and engagement, energy levels, processing speed, emotional regulation (Chapter 4, pp. 54-57), memory and self-regulation, when considering attentional control. Distraction in young children is mostly due to reduced sustained attention capacity and environmental distractions. Distraction in adolescents is more often due to decreased motor control/need to move and increased impulsivity (Hoyer et al., 2021). SLC skills and classroom learning strategies may therefore all be improved by targeting attention processes (see end of chapter on guidance for adaptive teaching), by considering and managing environmental stimuli (Hayden and Jordan, 2024), and by building in regular physical movement breaks.

Listening

> ⓘ **CRITICAL QUESTIONS**
>
> You can listen like a blank wall or like a splendid auditorium where every sound comes back fuller and richer.
>
> Alice Duer Miller (1940)
>
> - Ponder this quote and what it means.
> - When do you listen like a blank wall or like a splendid auditorium?

- What difference do these contrasting approaches to listening make to the information we glean and to our experiences?
- Think of the CYP you work with:
  - In what activities do they listen like a blank wall?
  - In what activities do they listen like a splendid auditorium?
  - How can you use this information to increase their attention and listening?

Whereas hearing involves the perception of sounds (page 29), listening is a more active process in which we attend (or not) to information conveyed to us through our senses. While physiological responses to simple sounds in the central auditory system are largely mature by four years of age, behavioural responses in listening and auditory processing tasks remain immature in most children until around eight or nine years (Moore, 2012). The ability to separate out the voice we're trying to listen to from other noises is a skill which develops over time, meaning younger children need quieter conditions than older children do. Although it can be thought that listening skills develop naturally, Hayes (2016, p. 47) asks whether listening is caught (develops naturally) or taught. Our environments contribute significantly to how we listen and what we learn to attend to or filter out (Gov.uk, 2022; National Literacy Trust, 2022). Switch costs are a loss of efficiency associated with redirecting attention from one stimulus to another. These form part of auditory attention, which is the ability to select and decode relevant stimulus whilst ignoring concurrent, irrelevant stimulus. Switch costs are influenced by the complexity of auditory scenes, which involve interactions between multiple factors such as screen-based technology, background noise and verbal language/instructions.

ⓘ CRITICAL QUESTIONS

- What are the switch costs in your classroom/learning environment?
- What do these mean for your learners and their access of the teaching and learning material?

Listening skills can be taught, for example, following a cochlear implant (Cole and Flexer, 2020) and adapting environments, for example, by reducing sensory stimuli, can improve listening for the individual learner. However, a more directed therapeutic approach will sometimes be necessary because poor listening skills can be the result of impaired auditory processing. Auditory processing, at its simplest, can be defined as the decoding of auditory information sent along the auditory pathway in the central nervous system. It is a complex process involving different neural mechanisms and breakdown can occur at several levels (Dillon and Cameron, 2021). Auditory processing difficulties and Auditory Processing Disorder (APD), which present despite normal hearing abilities, will likely require specific, tailored intervention (Chapter 6, page 89). That is not to say explicitly building listening tasks/activities into your pedagogy is not valuable, since doing so will increase the listening skills – and hence access to learning – for all your pupils (see 'guidance for adaptive teaching' on pages 34-35).

Listening in a communicative sense is an active process of receiving and responding to spoken (and sometimes unspoken) messages. There are several types of listening:

- **Selective listening** is where listeners pay attention to some parts of a message and skim over or ignore other parts of a message. This can happen when the information load is so great the listener cannot process all of it (for example, in a stressful medical appointment) or fit the information into their frame of reference (less conscious responses) and sometimes as a behavioural response (a more conscious response).
- **Active listening**. CYP and their carers will often have much to say, given time and understanding. We therefore need to consider our own listening skills. In her article *"Slow listening. The ethics and politics of paying attention, or shut up and listen"* Grehan (2019) explains how we should be fully attuned to both what is being said and the way it is being said before we make any move to respond. This is like 'reading the room' – where we attend to all aspects of a communication, both verbal and non-verbal, so we respond to the person and situation and not just to words. This requires effort, with the listener attuning to the feelings, views and experiences of the speaker and paying attention to inference, whilst demonstrating unbiased acceptance.
- **Thoughtful listening** (Clark, 2023) upends our authoritative position as educators and can be experienced as uncomfortable, though if we listen carefully and thoughtfully, our pedagogy changes in that we become able to respond to learning alongside the learners by identifying and meeting them 'where they are', thus moving towards meaningful and accessible co-construction.

Sensory and environmental factors

It is important to rule out the presence of physical hearing impairment when a CYP is experiencing difficulties with attention and listening skills. The hearing system consists of conductive hearing (capturing sound) and sensorineural hearing (converting sound into signals the brain can understand). A conductive hearing impairment means sound cannot pass efficiently through the outer and middle ear into the inner ear. This is often caused by temporary blockages such as wax in the outer ear or fluid in the middle ear (glue ear or otitis media), causing fluctuations in hearing, though conductive hearing impairments can be permanent in some cases. Sensorineural hearing impairment means the difficulty is occurring in the inner ear, generally because the cochlea isn't working properly, which is permanent, though medical advances, including a cochlear implant, can circumvent this in many cases.

Other sensory issues can also be contributing, including hyper (heightened) or hypo (lowered) sensitivity to noise such as can be experienced in sensory processing difficulties.

Sensory processing difficulties involve challenges with 'grading' sensory input, resulting in over-responsivity, under-responsivity or sensory seeking, all of which impact on achieving a balanced emotional state (needed for optimal performance and interactions, Chapter 4). Sensory processing difficulties can also involve challenges in the qualitative processing of sensory stimuli leading to difficulties knowing what the stimulus is and where it is coming from (Hoffman et al., 2022).

Difficulties with both physical hearing and sensory processing are why it is so important to consider the learning environment. Providing a suitable sensory environment, where an optimal level and type of stimulation are combined, can make a significant contribution to how teaching and learning opportunities are experienced and accessed. This may mean:

- assessing levels of noise and distractions;
- sitting the learner in the most optimal position for seeing and hearing;
- breaking down content into small, processable 'chunks';
- giving time to process and repeating if necessary;
- using visual cues to augment auditory information; and
- being aware the impact that other sensory stimuli such as heat, and factors such as affect (emotion) and tiredness, can have on a learner's ability to attend, listen to and process specific content.

This is because when we are stressed, we are more likely to process information using parts of the brain involved with emotions and survival rather than areas of the brain responsible for complex learning, auditory decoding and language. Not being able to attend and listen and so be present in lessons and able to access content is, in turn, stressful. Maslow's Hierarchy of Needs (1943) recognises that lower-level needs (such as physiological comfort and safety) must be met for higher-level functions (such as learning and self-actualisation) to take place (see Figure 14.1 page 203). Attending to the classroom sensory environment is therefore an essential step in enhancing SLC skills and learning. Tools such as the Classroom Sensory Environment Assessment (Kuhaneck and Kelleher, 2018) enable classroom practitioners to identify the most impactful sensory experiences present in a given learning setting. In addition to addressing and reducing some stimuli, practitioners can then use strategies such as sensory circuits (Horwood, 2009, see further reading/resources on page 36) to help children regulate and organise their senses to achieve the optimum level of alertness required for effective learning.

Speech, language and communication (SLC) skills and their influence on attention and listening

So far, we have considered attention and listening skills as prerequisite skills for the development of speech, language, communication and learning. It is also important to recognise if learners cannot attend or don't understand what is being said, they will disengage much faster. Difficulties with SLC can therefore, in turn, influence attention and listening *in situ*. There is also a danger of attention and listening difficulties being interpreted as behavioural in origin, rather than because of difficulties accessing spoken or written content. Certainly, CYP with attention and listening difficulties may:

- appear to ignore you;
- have difficulty sitting still;
- talk when they should be listening;
- be unable to tell you what you have been talking about;
- not know what to do/follow peers to find out;
- have difficulty following instructions;
- be able to concentrate on one thing only;
- be easily distracted;
- not settle with one activity and instead flit from task to task.

How this is recognised and supported will have a direct impact on their self-esteem, identity, social interactions and relationships.

> ⑦ **CRITICAL QUESTIONS**
>
> Think of a child or young person you know that displays the features listed in the bullet points above.
>
> - What helped you understand why they are displaying these features?
> - What helped you support them in your learning environment?
> - What challenges were part of this and what might you need to learn/know more about to help you address these?
> - How might you engage the CYP in this process?

When attention and listening challenges are more likely to be present

'Glue ear', a common condition in childhood, causes fluctuating conductive hearing difficulties as well as ear discomfort and tinnitus, and can delay SLC development (Nice, 2023). CYP with glue ear may mishear when not looking at who is speaking, may experience difficulties hearing in a group, and may ask for things to be repeated. They may have periods of illness, and may require medical supervision to decide on any needed interventions or support.

Two children in every class of 30, or 7.58% of children, start school with a **Developmental Language Disorder** (DLD) (RCSLT, 2021). DLD replaces the terms 'specific language impairment/disorder' or 'developmental language impairment'. DLD can co-occur with other neurodevelopmental difficulties, and CYP with DLD will experience difficulties with auditory processing, listening, attention, memory and language processing, especially when lots of information is being given orally (see Chapter 7 for more detail).

In the UK, the prevalence of **ADHD** (Attention Deficit Hyperactivity Disorder) in adults is estimated at 3–4%, with a male-to-female ratio of approximately 3:1 (NICE, 2024). Differences in neurological function (how neurons send information through the brain and which areas of the brain are activated for tasks), structure (some brain areas are slightly smaller), and development (delayed maturation of the brain's frontal lobe) which are distinct from cognitive ability, contribute to hyperactivity, impulsivity and inattention.

Prevalence estimates for **autism** have increased, currently sitting at around 1% (WHO, 2023), with the male-to-female ratio being between 3:1 and 5:1, thought to be as a result of females being better at masking their difficulties and 'fitting in' with societal expectations. Although difficulties with social interaction and communication are central to autism, differences in how people with autism focus and experience and process sensory information mean attention and listening skill challenges are often present.

It is difficult to estimate the prevalence of CYP who have experienced **trauma**, which is when we experience very stressful, frightening or distressing events that are difficult to cope with or out of our control. CYP with traumatic stress develop reactions that persist and affect their daily lives after the events have ended. For instance, they may have needed to be hypervigilant and will have learned to focus on some factors in their environment more than others, and to rapidly shift to a heightened state of alertness when a threat is perceived. They may have difficulties focusing attention, and they may not listen or may ignore direction (Erdman et al., 2020; Wass, 2021).

Note: This list is not exhaustive or mutually exclusive, but understanding underlying reasons why attention and listening challenges are present can help you plan your approach and support.

SPOTLIGHT ON EMERGING DEBATES
New media and attention and listening

Advances in technology, including the simultaneous use of multiple electronic platforms, mean most of us are increasingly breaking our attention from what we are doing or thinking about to check our texts, messages, social media and emails. Adults averaged 150 seconds on any screen before switching to another screen in 2004, compared to an average of 75 seconds in 2012, with a further reduction to 47 seconds occurring between 2016 and 2021 (Mark, 2023). New media (mobile touchscreen devices or MTSDs) is relatively new, and although we know children are using MTSDs at an increasingly early age and for an increasing amount of time (Ofcom, 2024), empirical research on how CYP's use of them is affecting health and wellbeing, including attention and listening skills, is also relatively new (Wass, 2018).

Some studies identify an association between higher digital media use at a younger age and increased inattention and impulsiveness, lower executive functions in general, and lower self-regulation (Konok and Szöke, 2022). However, we do not know definitively that it is the technology *causing* the attention problems, since it could equally be that the CYP's difficulties with attention are driving their increased technology use (new media is designed to capture and hold our attention). Other studies have found certain platforms improve cognitive skills (Wass, 2018) and being able to switch attention and respond to the evolving environment could be an evolutionary advantage going forward.

What we do know is outdoor time can benefit attention and memory, physical development, self-regulation and reduce stress. Goldberg's research on outdoor learning, focus and on-task behaviour, found some children (those who had the worst on-task attention indoors) were on task for 46% longer outdoors (Goldenberg, 2024). This means creating calm learning environments that minimise distraction and noise, and which enable deep work (when we focus intensely on a single task for an extended period of time). Nature provides this and whilst not every setting has access to a forest school, all can provide increased outdoor opportunities, for instance, at register, snack or circle time, and walking between classrooms, and all can increase how much nature is incorporated into aspects of the curriculum and classroom.

 CASE STUDY

Judith, primary teacher, outdoor learning officer

Child A, aged 6, sat in the classroom at 9am, dazed, oblivious to the productivity of pupils around him, to the empty desk in front of him where his pencil case and workbook should have been, to the routine which had been the same now for six months or more. Child A had achieved GLD (good level of development) in Reception 18 months before. That was before he began playing video games well into the night/playing games on his parent's phones on his way to school.

Despite multiple conversations with parents when they admitted his increasing use of technology, the situation continued for several months. Drawing him out of his reverie was challenging and the quality of work he produced was poor compared with what he was capable of. However, his lack of energy and motivation meant completing basic tasks was a huge achievement.

The honesty of his school report finally hit home. Child A's parents were shocked that he couldn't follow simple instructions or complete tasks in class without support to focus his attention and that he was at risk of not meeting the expected standard because of his impaired listening. Finally, the parents began closely monitoring and reducing his screen time – a battle at first but a positive change in the quality of his work meant his educational achievement got back on track.

This experience motivated my becoming an outdoor learning officer as I wanted to counter-act the increasing use of technology by CYP, help them re-connect with nature, and experience the health and well-being benefits of being outdoors. I've witnessed pupils, including those with ASD, ADHD and DLD being highly engaged and interacting with the natural environment in a way that has surprised their regular educators. For some, the outdoor environment is much calmer. Imagine a hall full of children vs a field/woodland area with the same number of children – it's much easier to focus on an activity or task when the noise isn't echoing all around you.

I believe that now, more than ever, educators should provide opportunities for children to experience the benefits of being outdoors. Whether this be 15 minutes at story time or longer sessions exploring the curriculum, I will continue to advocate the benefits for all, but especially for those children who find listening and attention easier in this environment.

ⓘ Critical questions

- How would you have responded to the scenario described above?
- How do you counteract the increasing levels of technology children are experiencing?
- How could you incorporate some outdoor time into your classroom routine?

GUIDANCE FOR ADAPTIVE TEACHING

Classroom practice activities which can help develop listening skills:

- Consider, and reduce, the levels of noise and auditory distractions present in your classroom environment.
- Precede the giving of instructions with an attention - gaining routine or sound sequence.

- Notice and make time for listening and understanding during everyday interactions.
- Check pupils' listening and understanding by asking them to repeat back what you have said – or to identify one or two keywords/points.
- Build opportunities for children to listen within curriculum content, e.g. by building up sound banks such as those on **Listening skills – BBC Teach** (https://www.bbc.co.uk/teach/school-radio/articles/zbc4y9q) (accessed 6 January 2025), using audio resources such as songs and audio stories, or playing simple games such as echo games, listening moments, musical statues or Chinese whispers.

Ten tips for effective listening (useful for both learner and teacher)

1) Face the speaker whenever possible.
2) Pay close attention and listen for ideas – find areas of interest to connect and attend to content, not delivery.
3) Don't interrupt and be patient.
4) Hold back your points or counterpoints – think about listening twice as much (we have two ears) as you speak (we have one mouth).
5) Resist distractions – stay in the moment.
6) Pay attention to non-verbal information.
7) Keep your mind open and be flexible to where the interaction might go.
8) Ask questions during pauses and demonstrate and check your listening by repeating what the listener has said.
9) Listen with empathy to try and see the speaker's viewpoint.
10) Provide instructions in written as well as verbal format, use meaningful visuals and present information in small 'chunks'.

CHAPTER SUMMARY

Attention and listening abilities underlie the development of SLC skills, as well as learning and achievement. Increased knowledge and understanding of how these develop and when/how difficulties with attention and listening might appear can help equip practitioners to more easily recognise, assess, support and seek help for the CYP under their care. This could be increasingly important as we consider, and seek to meet, challenges posed by new media.

Further reading/resources

Developing Minds: Attention and Concentration Challenges in Children and Young People – Developing Minds (accessed 6 January 2025).

- Includes sections on minimising distractions, building quick refocusing of attention, and working memory strategies.

Horwood, J (2009) *Sensory Circuits: A Sensory Motor Skills Programme for Children*, 3rd Edition. Hyde: LDA.

- A 10–15 minute plan of physical activities, consisting of alerting activities, organising activities and calming activities to enable children to achieve an optimal level of alertness.

Wass, S (2018) https://www.ted.com/talks/sam_wass_smarter_but_more_stressed_how_the_modern_world_is_changing_children (accessed 6 January 2025).

- This TED talk considers how features of the 21st century influences brain development, concentration, stress and learning capacities.

Wass, S and Goldenberg G (2025) *Take Action on Distraction*. London: Bloomsbury Publishing.

- A guide to improving attention and focus. Whilst aimed at the Early Years and Key Stage 1, you can creatively adapt the detail for other ages and stages.

References

Brown, T E (2006) Executive functions and attention deficit hyperactivity disorder: Implications of two conflicting views. *International Journal of Disability, Development, and Education*, 53(1): 35–46.

Clark, A (2023) *Slow Knowledge and the Unhurried Child: Time for Slow Pedagogies in Early Childhood Education*. Abingdon: Routledge.

Cole, E and Flexer, C (2020) *Children with Hearing Loss: Developing Listening and Talking: Birth to Six*. 4th Edition. Portland, OR: Plural Publishing.

Cooper, J, Moodley, M, and Reynell, J (1978) *Helping Language Development: A Developmental Programme for Children with Early Language Handicaps*. London: Edward Arnold.

Dillon, H and Cameron, S (2021) Separating the causes of listening difficulties in children. *Ear and Hearing*, 42(5): 1097–1108, https://doi.org/10.1097/AUD.0000000000001069

Erdman, S, Colker, L J, and Winter, E C (2020) *Trauma and Young Children: Teaching Strategies to Support and Empower*. Washington, DC: National Association for the Education of Young Children.

Goldenberg, G (2024) Outdoor learning, focus and on-task behaviour. *Instagram*, 24 January. Available at: Gemma Goldenberg (@phd_and_three) • Instagram photos and videos (https://www.instagram.com/p/C2feF7hsyx9/?img_index=1) (accessed 12 March 2025).

Gov.uk (2022) Help for early years providers: Listening and understanding (education.gov.uk) (accessed 12 March 2025).

Grehan, H (2019) Slow listening: The ethics and politics of paying attention, or shut up and listen. *Performance Research*, 24(8): 53–58.

Hayden, S and Jordan, E (2024) *Language for Learning in the Primary School: A Practical Guide for Supporting Pupils with Speech, Language and Communication Needs Across the Curriculum*. Abingdon: Routledge.

Hayes, C (2016) *Language, literacy & communication in the early years: a critical foundation*. Northwich: Critical Publishing Ltd.

Hoffman, D, Tomassi, R and Soares N (2022) Sensory processing difficulties. *International Journal of Child Health and Human Development*, 15(3): 275–287.

Horwood, J (2009) *Sensory Circuits: A Sensory Motor Skills Programme for Children*, 3rd Edition. Hyde: LDA.

Hoyer, R S, Elshafei, H, Hemmerlin, J, Bouet, R, and Bidet-Caulet, A (2021) Why are children so distractible? Development of attention and motor control from childhood to adulthood. *Child Development*, 92(4): e716–e737.

Konok, V and Szöke, R (2022) Longitudinal associations of children's hyperactivity/inattention, peer relationship problems and mobile device use. *Sustainability*, 24: 8845, https://doi.org/10.3390/su14148845

Kuhaneck, M H and Kelleher, J (2018) The classroom sensory environment assessment as an educational tool for teachers. *Journal of Occupational Therapy Schools & Early Intervention*, 11(2): 161–171 https://doi.org/10.1080/19411243.2018.1432442

Mark, G (2023) *Attention Span: Finding Focus for a Fulfilling Life*. London: William Collins.

Maslow, A H (1943) A theory of motivation. *Psychological Review*, 50: 370–396.

Miller, A D (1940) *The White Cliffs*. New York: Coward-McCann

Mirsky, A F, Anthony, B J, Duncan, C C, Ahern, M B, and Kellam, S G (1991) Analysis of the elements of attention: A neuropsychological approach. *Neuropsychology Review*, 2: 109–145.

Moore, D R (2012) Listening difficulties in children: Bottom-up and top-down contributions. *Journal of Communication Disorders*, 45(6): 411–418.

National Literacy Trust (2022) Speaking and listening National Literacy Trust (accessed 12 March 2025).

NICE (National Institute for Health and Care Excellence) (2023) *Otitis media with effusion in under 12s*. Available at: https://www.nice.org.uk/guidance/ng233 (accessed 12 March 2025).

NICE (National Institute for Health and Care Excellence) (2024) *Attention Deficit Hyperactivity Disorder*. Available at: Attention deficit hyperactivity disorder|Health topics A to Z | CKS | NICE (https://cks.nice.org.uk/topics/attention-deficit-hyperactivity-disorder/) (accessed 12 March 2025).

Ofcom (2024) *Children and Parents: media use and attitudes report 2024*. Childrens Media literacy report 2024 (ofcom.org.uk; https://www.ofcom.org.uk/__data/assets/pdf_file/0025/283048/Childrens-Media-Literacy-Report-2024.pdf) (accessed 12 March 2025).

RCSLT (Royal College of Speech and Language Therapists) (2021) *Giving Voice to People with Developmental Language Disorder*. Available at: rcslt-dld-factsheet.pdf (https://www.rcslt.org/wp-content/uploads/2021/10/rcslt-dld-factsheet.pdf) (accessed 12 March 2025).

Wass, S V (2018) *Smarter but More Stressed: How The Modern World Is Changing Children*. TED Talk. Available at: https://www.ted.com/talks/sam_wass_smarter_but_more_stressed_how_the_modern_world_is_changing_children (accessed 12 March 2025).

Wass, S V (2021) The origins of effortful control: How early development within arousal/regulatory systems influences attentional and affective control. *Developmental Review*, 61: 100978. https://doi.org/10.1016/j.dr.2021.100978

WHO (World Health Organisation) (2023) *Autism*. Available at: https://www.who.int/news-room/fact-sheets/detail/autism-spectrum-disorders (accessed 12 March 2025).

3 Play and conceptual development
Tom Hopkins

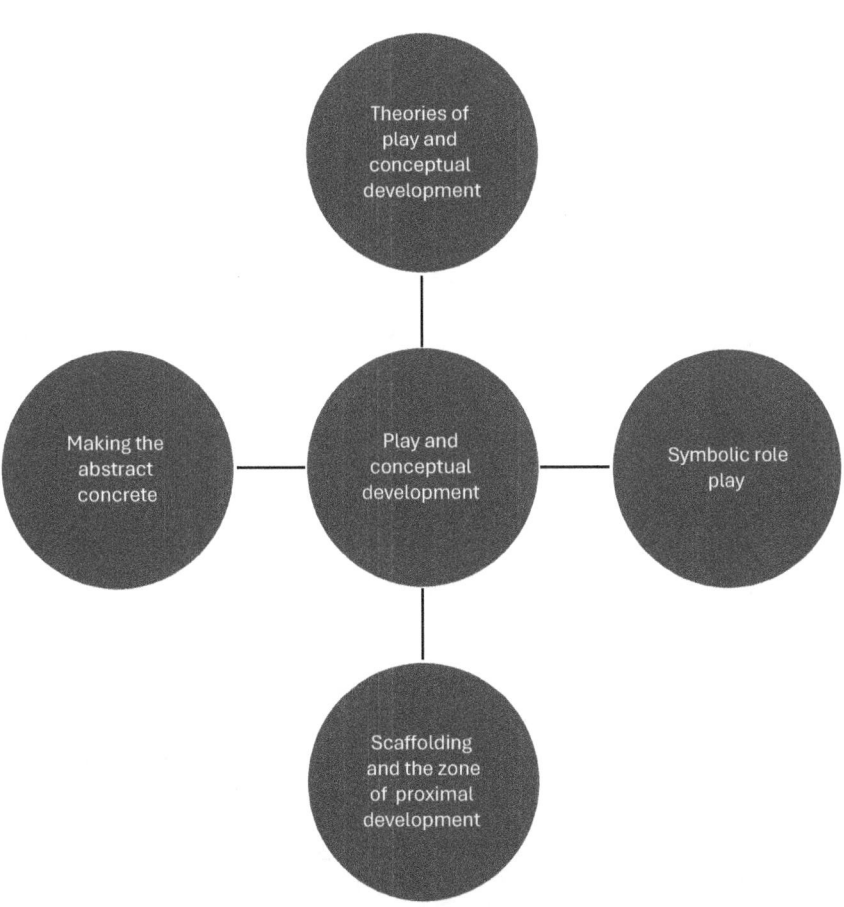

CHAPTER OBJECTIVES

Conceptual understanding is central to the development of a child's language, communication and overall learning. The inclusion of play in teaching can facilitate all of the above.

This chapter:

- explores theories that offer explanation of how concepts are learned and stored in memory;
- explains how explorative, object and symbolic role play uniquely contribute to the learning of concepts;
- identifies the importance of social interaction in play for the learning of concepts;
- provides educators with practical strategies and tips for how best to include play in their teaching of concept.

STARTING POINTS

- What type of concepts do you teach to your learners?
- How do you go about trying to help your learners understand these concepts?
- What do you notice works when you attempt this and what barriers or challenges do you face?
- How much play do you think you include in your teaching of concepts and do you think there is scope for more of this?

Introduction

Conceptual understanding is the symbolic representation of objects and events and the label attached to these. Concepts can be concrete and tangible in form, such as a 'car', or abstract in form, like 'love'. We refer to concepts through our communication with others, making conceptual understanding essential for language development (Nelson et al., 2014).

Play contributes to children's knowledge of concepts through different means. Children can learn the meaning of referents in their environment through independent explorative play with objects as well as through playful interactions. By engaging in playful scenes that incorporate 'pretend', and with the inclusion of characters/roles, learners can expand their language and their understanding of concepts. This is especially the case when educators create and scaffold opportunities for play that provide relatable narratives for learning concepts, including those considered abstract, that form core components of the curriculum. Play-based interventions should therefore be included in education for learners of all ages and must be adapted accordingly.

Theoretical explanations of concept development

The development of concepts (particularly concrete concepts) can be explained via mapping theory that illustrates how learners combine perceptual information about a referent they are attending to (Bloom, 2000). This information can include what the referent looks like, what it sounds like and what it does (its function) as well as the phonological information relating to the label of the referent that is often provided at the same time of exposure. The mapping of all these perceptual features can help learners to determine the meaning of the referent. After several instances of exposure, learners form a *prototype* (average) of this object that is stored in long-term memory and can be retrieved in instances where the object is referred to without it being physically present. Being exposed to the concept through multiple, various contexts will deepen a learner's knowledge of the prototype (Bloom, 2000).

Models from cognitive psychology illustrate how concepts are stored in long-term memory with similar related concepts situated together in a vast web or network of concepts (Singleton & Shulman, 2020). On repeat exposure to a known concept and/or its perceptual features, the relevant (assuming correct encoding) phonological and semantic features are 'fired up' or activated in the semantic memory network with any irrelevant information inhibited from activation. The more cues that are activated and inhibited as a result of mapping, the more efficient successful recall will be (Singleton & Shulman, 2020).

These concepts are stored in a hierarchal manner with basic concepts (dog) sitting underneath superordinate concepts (mammal) but above subordinate concepts (labrador). Learners are more likely to encounter basic ordinate concepts through their initial educational experience and thus need good understanding of these before being introduced to the more specific subordinate and the more general superordinate concepts that are prevalent in academic subjects (Beck et al., 2002; see Chapter 7 for more detail). However, research has shown the introduction of the latter in pre-school is related to increases in inductive reasoning skills since it encourages learners to find patterns amongst a category of different basic concepts (Suffill et al., 2022).

For the successful learning of concepts, educators should consider what pupils already know and what scope pupils have for expanding on this knowledge with support. Theoretically speaking, this process would be identifying the pupil's zone of proximal development (ZPD), (Vygotsky, 1987) and would require educators to therefore identify appropriate concepts that fall within this zone and not outside it (beyond pupils' capability). Once this is identified, educators can seek to 'scaffold' pupils to develop their knowledge of concepts through various strategies (see teaching concepts and guidance for adaptive teaching, p. 42).

The development of symbolic prototypes can be challenging for abstract concepts that are less concrete or tangible. Compared to the processing of concrete concepts that evoke both linguistic and pictorial mental images, there is an over reliance on linguistic features for the processing of abstract concepts (Sadoski, 2005). This can partly explain why learners are more likely to understand and learn concrete abstracts before those that can be considered to be more abstract in form, in which learners may need to draw on their developing social cognitive abilities (Bergelson & Swingley, 2013).

Note that it is still important for pupils to be introduced to basic concepts related to emotion (i.e. sad, angry) early in their education, given the importance that this has for supporting emotional regulation, self-awareness and empathy (Department for Education, 2024; see Chapter 11).

TEACHING CONCEPTS

Here are some suggestions that might help you in establishing a pupil's ZPD and to then scaffold their understanding of concepts for pupils of all ages:

Establish the core concepts. Consider what you want your learners to understand by the end of the session.

Work backwards from this 'core concept' to establish more basic concepts that underlie it and that are central to the foundations of the core concept. An example might be supporting learners to understand the concepts *floating* and *sinking* without the need to refer to *mass, density* and/or *gravity* (See Butts et al., 1993). For younger learners it could be targeting the concept *tall* before *taller*.

Provide concrete opportunities to demonstrate these basic concepts (see CPA method below) using examples that relate to a learner's everyday life and socio-cultural routine.

Provide explicit instructions that name the concept and that demonstrate its features and functions. Repeat this across varied contexts, including the concept within different sentences.

On successful learning of several basic concepts, consider *introducing the superordinate concept* that relates to all of the examples studied, highlighting their perceptual and semantic similarities.

Core curriculum subjects, such as maths and science encompass an abundance of abstract concepts, which some pupils find difficult to learn. The concrete, pictorial, abstract (CPA) approach developed initially by Bruner (1966), is widely used in education to support pupils' understanding of abstract concepts.

CONCRETE, PICTORIAL, ABSTRACT (CPA) APPROACH

Concrete:

> Provide concrete examples using physical materials that learners encounter in daily life to demonstrate conceptual knowledge;
>
> Provide explicit instruction to learners as they play with the physical materials and manipulate them to produce the desired concept (folding up a piece of paper in different ways to demonstrate *half*).

Pictorial:

> Once learners grasp the concrete stage, provide learners with instruction using pictorial images (diagrams that represent the varied ways of folding/cutting a paper in half).

Abstract:

> When learners are able to use pictures successfully, you can refer to more abstract symbols to represent the concept in teaching instruction such as the word 'half/halve' and the mathematical symbol '½'.

⑦ CRITICAL QUESTIONS

- What concepts are vital for your learners to understand? What other related concepts do you think your learners need to know to first?
- How could you try and make the teaching of these concepts more accessible, e.g. using visuals?

Play, conceptual development and the importance of symbolism

There is no standard definition of play, but common themes are reported that refer to it as an engaging and meaningful activity that learners of all ages enjoy participating in on a voluntary basis (Parker et al., 2022). There are also varying types of play, such as object/exploratory play, social play, symbolic play, role play and games with rules. Infants will demonstrate the first examples of play through their manipulation of objects until they begin to imitate short scenes that reflect episodes situated within their own lives (Casby, 2003). The benefits of play are widely reported to support learners in the development of their physical, cognitive, social and emotional wellbeing. It is therefore, considered a human right that all children should be provided with opportunities to play

(United Nations, 1989), and play theorists argue that play must therefore be embedded throughout the curriculum (Parker et al., 2022).

Play can support the development of concepts in different ways that complement the varied pedagogical theories of child development. Piagetian theory (1955) draws attention to the cognitive development that takes place in learners as they independently interact with their environment, constructing knowledge through a process of building upon and altering existing knowledge about their world (i.e. schema). It is through the learner's own playful exploration and experience of their world that conceptual knowledge is formed.

Piaget (1955) and Vygotsky (1987) emphasised the importance of acquiring symbolic thought (conceptual understanding) for language, which supports the association reported between symbolic play (pretend play) and language (Quinn et al., 2018). Symbolic play includes a combination of symbolic rituals (or scenes) that have been shown to correlate with the production of multi-word utterances in learners. It is argued that through symbolic play, learners are having to consider the conventional features and properties of the concept in addition to those that are being offered in the play scene, requiring multi-symbolic comparison/relations that have been shown to correlate with multi-word use (Shore, 1986). Pupils begin to display pretend play from around 18 months and are likely to replicate typical everyday rituals/actions that contain reference to everyday concepts onto themselves (putting themselves to sleep) before then doing so to others (like dolly or caregiver). From two years, learners are likely to refer to character emotions and desires (an example of how symbolic play can also support concepts of emotion) in short narrative scripts that reflect reality. They may also refer to items that aren't visible in the play scene or pretend an object is something other than what it is. At around 5–6 years, play scenes contain longer narrative sequences related to concepts that are manipulated and experimented with (Casby, 2003).

 HOW TO PROMOTE PLAY

In adherence to both Piagetian and the Montessori approach to play (Bienen, 2017), educators should facilitate an environment that encourages pupils to explore independently. They should provide a range of toys and activities that promote a multi-sensory experience that supports the development of fine/gross motor skills, problem-solving and language. Examples for the younger pupils include soft play, building blocks, playdough, waterplay and sandpit activities. For older pupils, taking trips out to parks, museums or farms, for example, can provide the same opportunities for playful learning.

Educators should use toys or play resources that reflect the learner's culture to encourage the re-enactment of familiar playful scripts that will incorporate known concepts. These could include objects in the natural environment: dolls, kitchen set ups and dress up clothes. Including neutral toys, such as Lego or blocks, is more likely to promote social play as well as symbolic play, based on that fact that they do not possess any obvious function that might limit the scope for imaginary play (Trawick-Smith et al., 2015).

The social side of play and its role in conceptual development

Play is culturally specific and therefore diverse. The opportunities provided to children for the various forms of play reflect unique cultural values that include child-rearing practices which contribute to the acquisition of culturally specific concepts (Vygotsky, 1987). For example, children of indigenous communities situated in remote parts of South America, are encouraged to play freely, unsupervised in their natural environment in line with their views of how children develop (Gosso et al., 2018). Families in collectivist cultures in Asia, favour play that involves physical touch and encourages interpersonal connection, whereas in Western, industrialised cultures there is more of a focus on verbal exchanges with objects (Roopnarine et al., 2018).

Interactionist perspectives of language acquisition emphasise the importance of the socio-cultural context (Singleton & Shulman, 2020). It argues that conceptual knowledge is developed through the communication and language that is embedded within socio-cultural routines and playful practice, which themselves are afforded, modelled and scaffolded by experts in the pupils' environment (Vygotsky, 1987).

In Western culture, examples of this occur in the early years setting through playful routines that incorporate joint attention to objects in a learner's environment. Joint attention involves the sharing of an experience that all communicative partners are aware of and is a strong predictor of vocabulary development due to the communicative intent involved (Tomasello et al., 2007). Episodes of joint attention often contain communicative intent modelled by caregivers through verbal means and non-verbal gesture, which the learners learn to imitate once they realise the effect they can have on their communicative partner. In fact, play can also support learners in making this realisation through predictable games like 'peek-a-boo' or 'ready-steady-go'! Playful routines like peek-a boo can also support turn-taking; an important feature of conversation (Singleton & Shulman, 2020). Play routines that include joint attention and communicative intent can also support a learner's understanding of more abstract concepts like '*all gone*'. In fact, by making a point of searching for a specific object and naming the intent with phrases such as '*where is the ball?*', the concept of ball and other associated concepts (i.e. where) become salient to learners when the adult after finding the ball points to it and expresses joy in doing so: *There's the ball!*

> **HOW TO SUPPORT CONCEPTUAL DEVELOPMENT THROUGH JOINT ATTENTIVE PLAY**
>
> *Allow time* for the learners to initiate communication either through gesture or vocalisation.
>
> Provide a *joyful* and *engaging* environment that promotes independent exploration.
>
> →

> *Follow the child's lead* and attention rather than directing the child's attention as you are more likely to experience a successful episode of joint attention and a shared communication exchange with something that the child wants to play with or is inquisitive about exploring.
>
> *Provide a running commentary* on what the pupil is doing to provide a model of concepts that the pupil can refer to.
>
> *Respond* to the learners once they have initiated the exchange and direct your response to the activity that the learner is engaging in or wants to as a way of acknowledging their communicative intent. Again, it is important to allow time for the learners to respond to model effective turn-taking.

Using role play to support the development of concepts

Role play can be used for pupils of all ages with more advanced forms used for older pupils in class activities that promote the understanding of abstract concepts that relate to the curriculum. Role playing scenes that resemble typical life experiences has been shown to improve conceptual knowledge of target vocabulary for learners including those of an additional language (Alabsi, 2016). Blanchard and Buchs, (2015) found pupils reported a stronger understanding and interest in the concept of sustainability after participating in a debate in character of a representative of an organisation that held a specific view of the concept. Pupils spent time preparing for the debate and opportunities for peer feedback were also provided which pupils responded to, adapting their speech accordingly. This activity also made them more aware of their interpersonal skills. A debriefing session allowed learners to summarise what they had learned on the concept from the activity and gave teachers the opportunity to provide guidance and feedback on points expressed and or missed. Role play enables learners to have fun and play around with concepts and language in a safe space that promotes engagement and motivation. Gamification is another example of how play can achieve this in the learning of concept through the application of games with rules that creates a competitive reward-based learning activity aligned to specific learning objectives for pupils of all ages (Zeybek & Saygı, 2024).

 CASE STUDY

Andy, 41, secondary school English teacher

I have found that some learners, particularly those with educational needs, can find Shakespeare difficult to engage in not just for the accessibility, but also the relevance it has to their lives. For the opening scene of Romeo and Juliet, I decided to incorporate improvised role play to engage learners in the key concept of conflict related to the text, providing learners with the opportunity to replicate their own versions of the scene.

After learners were familiar with the scene, I arranged them into small groups and prompted them to consider an opening line that could initiate different versions of conflict. We would also highlight patterns in the wording of these opening lines, with reference to emotion and intent. When the groups had an opportunity to run through their scenes, I asked the learners how these characters might feel and they came up with a range of emotions, such as anger, rage, jealousy, fear, anxiety and bravery. I then assigned each group an emotion to incorporate into the original scene to see how they appeared physically in the original scene, relating them back to the beliefs and intentions of the main characters. As they did this, I also asked them how they thought these reactions were contributing to the conflict.

Next, as a whole group, we considered how the conflict could be resolved by Benvolio and Tybalt with the aim of collaboratively producing strategies that could be used to regulate emotion and manage conflict. They came up with examples like listening, trying to understand, showing empathy and disagreeing in a calm manner, and so on.

Finally, I asked all groups to re-enact one of the scenes they produced by trying to solve the conflict using these strategies to demonstrate this in action. As homework afterwards, I created a sheet that prompted learners to reflect on emotion in conflict, how it can be represented by language and how this emotion could be managed through different types of language.

By incorporating improvised role play in the study of concepts via Shakespeare, learners were given the opportunity to create a scene that they could relate to, and flexibly adapt to add meaning to what was an abstract concept. I found that not only did this increase engagement but also self-confidence for learners who wouldn't usually contribute in class.

ⓘ Critical questions

Consider how Andy identified key concepts in his teaching of Shakespeare and how he incorporated play in providing learners with the opportunity to explore their knowledge of these.

- What lessons can you take away for your own practice?

- How could you incorporate role play in your practice to promote a fun engaging learning environment.

- How could you use play to provide a learning platform that builds on concepts and life experience familiar to your learners.

- How might you balance a structured approach that aligns to clear learning objectives to one that allows learners the freedom to create their own role play.

SPOTLIGHT ON EMERGING DEBATES

There is still some debate over the extent to which learners are able to apply what they have learned about concepts through free play or whether more guided, explicit instruction is required for them to fully understand concepts (Disney & Li, 2022). By enabling children to initiate and create their play world, educators can attend and collaborate with them on play scripts that children are emotionally invested in. Educators can guide exploration; support problem-solving and embed conceptual knowledge/instruction to the play episode. Educators should be dynamic in how much support and explicit instruction is required from them depending on the pupils' knowledge (Disney & Li, 2022).

GUIDANCE FOR ADAPTIVE TEACHING

Considerations for the teaching of concepts in play (Based on Nelson et al., 2014)

Isolation: Initial exposure of the target concept should occur separately to other concepts so that only one interpretation of the concept can be made. By introducing the colour blue, you would need to take into account anything else about the blue object that is being shown to the chid (i.e. the shape). So ensuring that shape remains constant (i.e. using different coloured circles) would be important here to ensure that children are primed to encode the word blue as referring only to the colour of the object.

Positive examples: After initial exposure, you can begin to introduce different variants of the concept to allow for generalisation. These other examples should share key features of the target concept that lie on a spectrum, so showing them different birds including a robin, eagle and ostrich, for example.

Offer alternative non-examples: Offer alternative examples that do not represent the target concept. Try and keep all other features of the example constant where possible to avoid confusion and to help guide learners' attention to key features that can be used to build the prototype. An example could be introducing the concept *under* by positioning a Lego person under a Lego bridge. This can be compared with the non-example of over the bridge using the same Lego person and bridge. It is also advised that the non-example is one that can be considered to be very different to the target concept. The non-example should also be examples of concepts that learners already know so as not to introduce another novel concept to them at the same time.

Narrate what the learner is doing whilst making reference to specific terminology that includes and relates to the concept of study.

Ask open questions to the learners as they perform the tasks as a way to establish their knowledge of the concept.

Offer opportunities for expansion through the testing of new questions/hypothesis that learners should be prompted to consider via additional experimentation and demonstration.

Reflect on what was learned to allow time for consolidation of the key aspects and features of the concept.

Engelmann & Carnine (1982) suggest that within a 20-minute session, there could be an opportunity to focus on 6–8 positive examples of a concept along with a similar number of non-examples.

CHAPTER SUMMARY

Play has many benefits for learner development, including language, and should therefore be included in teaching activities across the ages and the curriculum. Educational staff should be supported in doing so, provided with time, resources and training to enable play to be incorporated effectively in school education. Learners should be supported to access the abstract through play and provided with the opportunity to create play scenes that explore these concepts in detail to deepen their understanding. This is particularly important when instances of pretend symbolic play in learner's lives is slowly decreasing (Howes & Wishard, 2004).

Further reading/resources

Exploring Words – Help for Early Years Providers https://help-for-early-years-providers.education.gov.uk/areas-of-learning/literacy/exploring-words

Helping Children Learn New Words: Early Years – Speech and Language UK: Changing Young Lives: https://speechandlanguage.org.uk/educators-and-professionals/resource-library-for-educators/helping-children-learn-new-words-early-years/

The Word Gap: The Early Years Make the Difference | NAEYC https://www.naeyc.org/resources/pubs/tyc/feb2014/the-word-gap

Using Early Childhood Classroom Activities to Build Vocabulary. https://www.hanen.org/information-tips/using-early-childhood-classroom-activities-to-build-vocabulary

References

Alabsi, T A (2016) The effectiveness of role play strategy in teaching vocabulary. *Theory and Practice in Language Studies*, 6(2): 227–234.

Beck, I L, McKeown, M G, and Kugan, L (2002) *Bringing Words to Life*. New York: Guilford Press.

Bergelson, E and Swingley, D (2013) The acquisition of abstract words by Young infants. *Cognition* 127(3): 391–397.

Bienen, H (2017) *The Montessori Method*. 1st edition. [Online]. London: Taylor & Francis Group.

Blanchard, O and Buchs, A (2015) Clarifying sustainable development concepts through role-play. *Simulation and Gaming*, 46(6): 697–712.

Bloom, P (2000) *How Children Learn the Meanings of Words*. 1st ed. Cambridge, MA: MIT Press.

Bruner, J S (1966) *Toward a Theory of Instruction*. Cambridge, MA: Harvard University Press.

Butts, D P, Hofman, H M, and Anderson, M (1993) Is hands-on experience enough? A study of young children's views of sinking and floating objects. *Journal of Elementary Science Education*, 5(1): 50–64.

Casby, M W (2003) The development of play in infants, toddlers and young children. *Communication Disorders Quarterly*, 24(4): 163–174.

Department for Education (2024) Early years foundation stage statutory framework for group and school-based providers. Available at: https://assets.publishing.service.gov.uk/media/670fa42a30536cb92748328f/EYFS_statutory_framework_for_group_and_school_-_based_providers.pdf (Accessed: 23rd January 2025).

Disney, L and Li, L (2022) Above, below, or equal? Exploring teachers' pedagogical positioning in a playworld context to teach mathematical concepts to preschool children. *Teaching and Teacher Education*, 114, 103706.

Engelmann, S., and Carnine, D (1982) *Theory of instruction: Principles and Applications*. New York: Irvington Publishers.

Gosso, Y, Resende, B D, and Carvalho, A M A (2018) Play in South American indigenous children. In Smith P K, and Roopnarine J L, (eds.). *The Cambridge Handbook of Play: Developmental and Disciplinary Perspectives*. Cambridge: Cambridge University Press, 322–342.

Howes, C and Wishard, A G (2004) Revisiting shared meaning: Looking through the lens of culture and linking shared pretend play through proto-narrative development to emergent literacy. In Zigler E, Singer D G, and Bishop-Josef, S J, (eds.). *Children's play: The Roots of Reading*. 1st edition. Washington, DC: Zero to Three Press, 143–158.

Nelson, L H, Powell, K L, and Bloom, S E (2014) Development of basic concepts in early education programs for children who are deaf and hard of hearing using listening and spoken language. *The Volta Review*, 114(1): 7–27.

Parker, R, Thomsen, B S, and Berry, A (2022) Learning through play at school: A framework for policy and practice, *Frontiers in Education* 7:751801.

Piaget, J (1955) *The Language and Thought of the Child*. M Gabain (Trans). Cleveland, OH: Meridian.

Quinn, S, Donnelly, S, and Kidd, E (2018) The relationship between symbolic play and language acquisition: A meta-analytic review. *Developmental Review*, 49(2): 121–135

Roopnarine, J L, Yildirim, E D, and Davidson, K L (2018) Mother-child and father-child play in different cultural contexts. In Smith, P K and Roopnarine, J L, (eds.). *The Cambridge Handbook of Play: Developmental and Disciplinary Perspectives*, Cambridge, MA: Cambridge University Press, 322–342.

Sadoski, M (2005) A dual coding view of vocabulary learning. *Reading & Writing Quarterly*, 21(3): 221–238.

Shore, C (1986) Combinatorial play, conceptual development, and early multiword speech. *Developmental Psychology*, 22(2): 184–190.

Singleton, N C and Shulman, B B (2020) *Language development: Foundations, Processes, and Clinical Applications*. 3rd edition. Burlington, MA: Jones & Bartlett Learning.

Suffill, E, Schonberg, C, Vlach, H A, and Lupyan, G (2022) Children's knowledge of superordinate words predicts subsequent inductive reasoning. *Journal of Experimental Child Psychology*, 221(1): 105449.

Tomasello, M, Carpenter, M, and Liszkowski, U (2007) A new look at infant pointing. *Child Development*. [Online] 78(3):705–722.

Trawick-Smith, J, Wolff, J, Koschel, M, and Vallarelli, J (2015) Effects of toys on the play quality of preschool children: Influence of gender, ethnicity, and socioeconomic status. *Early Childhood Education Journal*, 43(4): 249–256.

United Nations (1989) *Convention on the Rights of the Child*. General comment no 31. Available at: Convention on the Rights of the Child text|UNICEF [Accessed 13 March 2025].

Vygotsky, L S (1987) Thinking and speech. In Rieber R and Carton A. (eds.), L. S. *Vygotsky, Collected works*, Vol. 1:39–285. New York: Plenum.

Zeybek, N and Saygı, E (2024) Gamification in education: Why, where, when, and how? A Systematic Review *Games and Culture*, 19(2): 237–264.

4 Emotional regulation in the classroom

Helen Knowler

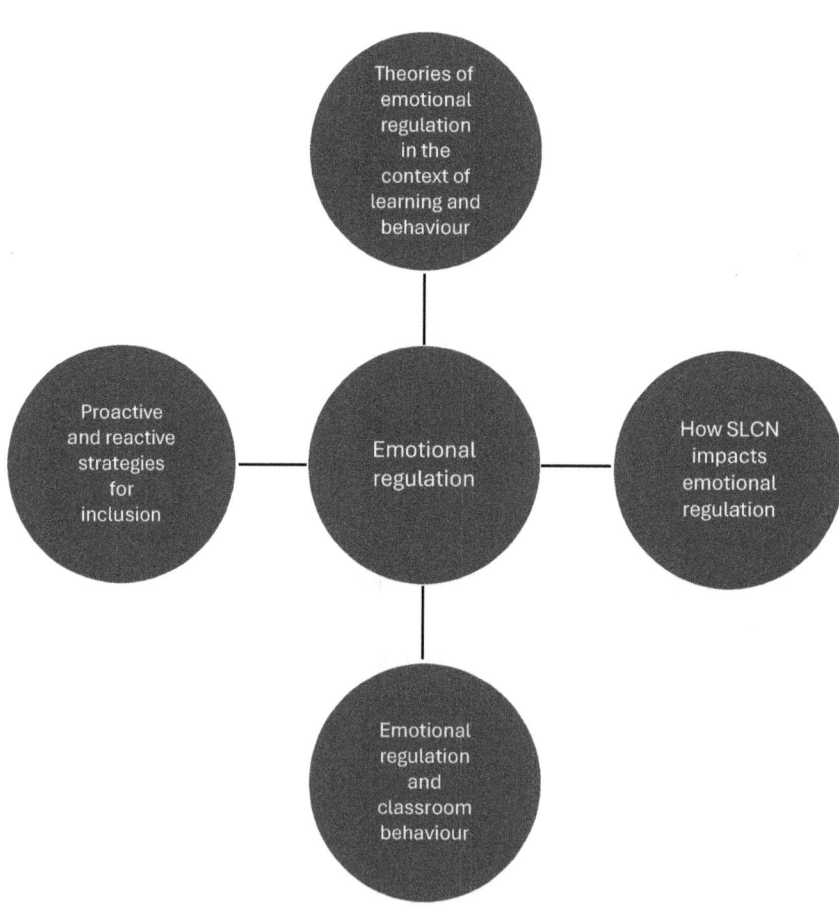

🎯 CHAPTER OBJECTIVES

This chapter explores the dynamic relationship between emotional regulation in the classroom, speech, language and communication needs (SLCN), and will give you ideas for developing your own toolkit of inclusive approaches to supporting learners. The chapter

- explores theories related to emotional regulation and learning and the ways SLCN can impact emotional regulation;
- uses critical questions to identify the key challenges supporting emotional regulation;
- identifies solutions and possibilities to cementing inclusive practice when developing knowledge and expertise in supporting emotional regulation.

Introduction

Positive mental health and wellbeing are a significant feature of inclusive classrooms and have been even more pertinent since the COVID-19 pandemic of 2020. Professionals who work in, and adjacent to, educational settings understand better the importance of healthy schools (Weare, 2013) in supporting social, emotional and academic achievement. One challenge with developing positive mental health and wellbeing is that we tend to get better at it as we get older because we have important opportunities to get over difficult emotional situations, try things out and experience successes. We are also more likely to have acquired the language to process and express these emotions.

Childhood and adolescence are substantive phases in the development of emotional regulation and are also times when we spend a lot of time in school. School settings and the people in them provide an important context for learning to develop emotional literacy skills (being able to understand one's own feelings and to empathise with the feelings of others in a way that enhances living (Steiner, 1997), develop positive relationships with adults and peers, and to learn how to manage when things go wrong. Ripley and Yuill (2005) argue that language competence is a key factor in developing emotional literacy, including self-regulation and relationships with peers and adults in a school community. While emotional dysregulation in schools can be upsetting and a serious barrier to inclusion, this chapter assumes that teachers, speech and language therapists (SaLTs) and other professionals can do a lot to improve communication before any psychological input is needed Chang and Taxer (2020). It is common to assume that better communications skills are needed to access help and support, but in fact having good communications skills in the first place is itself a protective factor for further or more significant mental health issues due to emotional dysregulation. Research in communication conditions (Hobson et al., 2019) such as alexithymia, a condition that makes it difficult to express and understand emotions, shows that simply talking itself can regulate and develop emotional responsiveness and thus reduce the impact of experiencing negative emotions.

> ⚑ **STARTING POINTS**
>
> - How do you understand emotional regulation in the context of your own classroom?
> - How do SLCN impact emotional regulation for learners?
> - In turn, what have you noticed can be effective in helping learners with SLCN to regulate their emotions when learning?
> - What are the implications for your own professional learning and development?

What is emotional regulation?

Emotional regulation is described as the ability to manage and change our emotions. It can also be defined as the ability to 'deal with feelings' or more formally to be able to 'process' how we feel when something has happened so we can return to the state we were before an emotion occurred. However, the ability to name or label an emotion is just the first step in the process of emotional regulation, and this is where we can see the potential of the educational setting and the role of education professionals as an important mechanism for the development of effective emotional regulation skills when at school. Emotional regulation can be a helpful term because it assigns no value (good or bad) to emotions and means we are less likely to label pupils as such, depending on the emotional state we see them in most often.

Whatever theories of emotion or language development we draw from in our practice, the role of language is crucial so that learners can reason, reflect and discuss emotions. The process model of emotional regulation demonstrates a sequence over time, whereby a learner experiences the following steps or stages and shows how the process of emotional regulation is dynamic, iterative and ongoing.

Figure 4.1 illustrates that a learner will experience a **situation** that is relevant and in a particular context. For this chapter, we would expect this to be a classroom or related space within an early years setting, school, college or university. In turn, this situation as it occurs is enough to warrant a learner's **attention** and would involve changing the learner's attention from whatever they are doing at that time towards a more emotional engagement. For example, a learner could be engaged in a task, but overhear a conversation that catches their attention, or they notice the task is getting harder to do. At this point, the learner will **appraise** or evaluate the situation usually from an instinctual and embodied perspective and finally an emotional **response** is generated. This response could be cognitive, behavioural, affective or physiological but will be mediated by previous experiences utilising existing skills and capabilities and experience of successful self-regulation. For some learners, this process will be incredibly quick and their experience and awareness of it will be imperceptible. The context will also play a significant role, since whether this process happens in a small and supported environment or large and

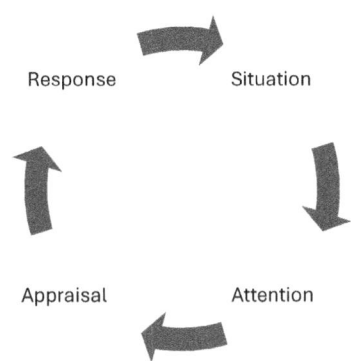

Figure 4.1 *The process model of emotional regulation*

busy classroom, there will be implications for how the learner behaves and whether there is a positive or negative consequence.

Emotional regulation depends on a range of skills and abilities and the key aim of any support or intervention is to help anyone who becomes emotionally dysregulated to become able to self-regulate in a way that is appropriate for a particular context. Co-regulation, where others support the regulation, may be required for children and young people not yet able to self-regulate. Core dimensions of supporting skills development include:

- **Understanding language**: vocabulary, grammar and instructions.
- **Emotional literacy skills**: labelling of own feelings and those of others and managing own emotions with words.
- **Inferencing and verbal reasoning**: 'reading between the lines' and working out what has not been explicitly stated (in conversation and reading) and verbalising one's own thinking.
- **Narrative skills**: describing real events, including one's own life story, but also fictional stories.
- **Social problem-solving**: using talk to think about how people interact with one another and how to sort out misunderstandings.

(Branagan, Cross and Parsons, 2020)

Language, emotion and emotional regulation in education

According to Hobson et al. (2019) most theories of emotions in humans suggest language mechanisms and processes contribute to our emotional responses to the world around us, although there is much debate and discussion around how this relationship is constituted. Research into emotional regulation in the UK, as an academic discipline, dates to the 1970s when leading researchers, such as Professor Sir Michael Rutter, began to explore the psycho-social development of children with communication challenges such as the relationship between developmental receptive language disorders and mental health. These research teams found significant evidence that children and young people who were identified as having SLCN were also at risk of developing social and emotional difficulties and mental health conditions later in life (Jagoe and Walsh, 2020). This work laid the path to our understanding of the role of emotion and emotional regulation in learning and that it is a crucial dimension a professional's role in facilitating the development of inclusive cultures in schools. It is fair to say the role of emotion and the capacity of educators to work with concepts of emotional regulation have not always been seen to be important or a priority for schools. For example, the development of social and emotional learning (SEL) programmes has not always been embraced by teachers, researchers and policymakers such as in the case of the roll-out of the Social and Emotional Aspects of Learning (SEAL) (DfE, 2010) programme in the early 2000s in England. Critiques of initiatives such as these, cite the challenges of incorporating SEL into a busy curriculum and the skills and expertise of teachers as significant issues. Additionally, Ecclestone and Hayes (2009) argue the rise of therapeutic education that these initiatives can foster is dangerous since it makes learners more anxious and can trigger dependency in learners that undermines learning and achievement. However, a counter argument is that these challenges to the importance of SEL and emotional regulation fail to take account of the experiences of learners with SLCN as whole people and are based on ableist notions of the 'ideal' child who presents no obstacles to curriculum delivery and can learn at a pace always set by the teacher.

There is now ample evidence (Jagoe and Walsh, 2020) that the ability to positively manage emotions and regulate emotions in the classroom space is essential for success and that those learners who can talk about their emotions and express themselves are often more likely to be 'school ready'. In turn, these learners can more effectively manage the various barriers and challenges they will face as a natural consequence of being at school.

Generally, theories of emotion and emotional regulation emphasise the ability to be able to recognise our emotions in an embodied sense (interoception) as well as a cognitive sense and then be able to articulate these feelings. While there are differing perspectives on language acquisition, under most accounts, language plays a crucial role in our ability to recognise and process emotions. Therefore, any kind of language difficulty, however small or insignificant, would seriously impact on a learner's ability to manage emotions in any context, not least the busy world of classrooms.

Binns et al. (2019) assert that at least half of learners with SCLN experienced challenges in recognising and managing emotions and reactions to the world around them. Apart from the obvious challenge that learning to talk about emotions is difficult for anyone, learners who struggle to be able to identify and talk about their emotions are at significant risk of exclusion and behaviour sanctions, while their inability to regulate emotions is seen as poor behaviour or rule breaking (see Chapters 11 and 13). Additionally, in Western cultures, we tend to have 'norms' around what are seen to be expected or healthy emotions in particular contexts. This means the adults supporting learners need to have a strong understanding of culturally appropriate responses to relationship building, for example, with learners who have SCLN and for whom English is not their first language Wren et al. (2023). It also means we must be critically reflective around the kinds of responses we encourage and teach learners, especially as they approach adolescence (see Chapter 12).

Emotional dysregulation and classroom behaviour

According to Lancastle et al. (2024) emotional dysregulation means some learners will experience challenges in:

- an **awareness and understanding of emotions** relevant and appropriate to age and context;
- **acceptance of emotions** as we experience and feel them in our daily lives;
- an **ability to engage in goal-directed behaviour** and avoid acting impulsively when experiencing negative emotions
- **access to emotion regulation strategies** perceived as effective by self and others.

This list of challenges makes it fairly clear how difficult it can be for any learner to practise and develop skills for emotional regulation, and given that school aged learners are generally between 4 and 18 years of age, it can be surprising to think how effective most children and young people are in school settings. Emotional dysregulation can manifest in many ways but according to Burden (2017) this could show up in the following ways:

- It is difficult to stop doing something when I know I shouldn't do it.
- People tell me that I get loud and wild when I get excited about something.
- If there are other things going on around me, I find it hard to keep my attention focused on whatever I'm supposed to be doing.
- I become upset when things don't go my way/the way I am expecting them to.
- When I'm bored, tired or upset I fidget and just can't sit still.
- It's hard for me to notice when I've had enough (sweets, sugary drinks, etc.).
- I find it difficult to wait.
- I get upset easily and feel like I can't cope.
- It is difficult for me to control my temper.

SPOTLIGHT ON EMERGING DEBATES

In 2023, the NHS published the results of the 'Mental Health of Children and Young People in England' survey (NHS, 2023) which showed that around one in five children and young people had a probable mental health issue. For 8- to 16-year-olds, the rates of probable mental health issues were similar for boys and girls and of this group, 26.8% had a parent who could afford to take their child to activities out of school. Those between 11 and 16 years of age with probable mental health issues, were five times more likely to have been bullied (36.9% compared to 7.6% of those without probable mental health issues). The survey also revealed the extent of concern among children and young people on issues such as climate change, economic stability and having enough money, and eating disorders, revealing that to be a child or young person in today's classrooms can be worrying and stressful. This also presents a challenge to professionals supporting learners in schools and other educational settings such as special schools or alternative provision (AP) because it blurs the lines of professional expectations. Whereas teachers may have traditionally considered their role to be about curriculum delivery, notions of curriculum have expanded considerably over the last twenty years so that teachers, teaching assistants and senior leaders in schools must consider a much wider range of factors that impact learning, behaviour and achievement Wren et al. (2023). It also means that it is no longer viable in an inclusive setting to say that emotional and pastoral support is not the role of educators and this can be seen in Oftsed's (2024) inspection framework encompassing evaluation of factors such as personal development, stating *'336.The curriculum provided by schools should extend beyond the academic, technical or vocational. Schools support pupils to develop in many diverse aspects of life'*.

This expansion of concerns for schools was bought into sharp relief during and after the pandemic when the sudden increase in e-learning and digital teaching methodologies became essential to keep schools open and learners engaged. Supporting and managing mental health and wellbeing during this time became very difficult but also exposed the ways that schools had not thought about the role of emotions and digital engagement. As Mayer (2020) points out, our understanding of the range of emotions learners experience while engaging in digital learning is limited. It also means that in thinking about emotional regulation, it is likely that strategies used for in-classroom/in-person support will need to be modified and adapted since digital and e-learning can often happen individually and in isolation. It is interesting to reflect on the role of the professional in supporting emotional regulation online or asynchronously when they cannot be there at the time or soon after an experience of dysregulation. As Mayer goes on to argue, there is a requirement to reconceptualise the identification of the range of emotions experienced in an e-learning context – and while progress is being made to understand this new dynamic for educators, learners will still need appropriate and timely support.

SUPPORTING AND ENHANCING EMOTIONAL REGULATION

There are many ways to support learners with SLCN to learn how to develop positive strategies for emotional regulation and, as outlined above in Figure 4.1, the dynamic nature of learning how to manage an emotional response means that learning can be supported by a wide range of strategies and approaches. Generally, when working with learners, the longer-term goal is to support independence in the regulation of emotion towards successful outcomes in the classroom. It is not realistic, or even desirable to aim to eliminate emotional dysregulation, and so a key challenge in terms of developing support rests on supporting learners to understand how to deal with emotions when they arise and not to rely on unrealistic expectations of eradicating emotions we consider to be negative. This can unwittingly develop into harmful 'zero tolerance' approaches to behaviour management, moving support away from the more inclusive cognitive-emotional direction of emotional regulation techniques. This example demonstrates how this can happen and shows how Sarjit worked with colleagues to support Jason.

CASE STUDY 1
Supporting Jason – initial support

Sarjit is an assistant SENCo in her primary school and has been enjoying working to develop strategies for learners to manage their anger and frustration when they find a task difficult. Jason is in year 5 and stammers, and can often become very explosive if he cannot finish a task at the same time as his peers. Sarjit has worked with Jason to understand that shouting, swearing and kicking chairs or tables is not a good way to manage his feelings. In the 1:1 session with the teaching assistant, Jason has been learning breathing techniques and how to take a break. To discourage Jason from using his 'old' techniques, Sarjit developed a system to give Jason three chances to practise and get his choices 'right'. She uses a colourful chart with dry wipe pens where Jason can keep track of his choices. If Jason makes a poor choice after three occasions, he will receive a sanction and be asked to leave the classroom.

In this case study, Sarjit has correctly identified that learners with a stammer regularly experience frustration in busy classrooms. Many learners will do as much as they can to hide their stammer and worry intensely about having to speak or read aloud. It also means that asking for help in a timely manner can be challenging for Jason and the physiological barrier of pronouncing and articulating phonemes (sounds) can be tiring and extremely distressing as learners experience blocks or repetitions. Stammering can also be experienced in conjunction with other conditions such as dyspraxia, ADHD or Tourette's syndrome. This means that learners can experience significant barriers to accessing the curriculum and can struggle to stay focused and motivated even if they find a topic interesting and stimulating. Sarjit discovered that despite her attempts to support Jason to see that his emotional outburst was not appropriate, she had focused too much on the presenting behaviours and not enough on supporting Jason to talk about how he felt about his anger and frustration. She reflected that she had focused on modifying problematic behaviours which meant that Jason soon realised that on some days he could reach the point of sanction literally within 5 minutes. Jason became frustrated and angry, and Sarjit began to see him as a naughty and problematic learner.

CASE STUDY 2
Supporting Jason – following reflection and reframing

Sarjit decided to talk to her SENCo and the SaLT that had been working with Jason. She explained her commitment to keeping Jason in the classroom and her interest in developing inclusive strategies. In the reflective dialogue between the three professionals, it became obvious that a reframing of the issue could have significant positive impacts for both Jason and Sarjit. Firstly, it was agreed that Sarjit could support Jason to feel relaxed and rather than offer a warning, a reminder to breathe and calm down should be the first things to do. Sarjit researched calming strategies and the use of objects and made Jason a 'calm down kit' which included a cushion, an egg timer, some fidget toys and a short booklet with breathing exercises. Sarjit worked closely with the SaLT and teaching assistant to develop activities based on the Window of Tolerance theory (Siegel, 1999), so that everyone could better understand Jason's capabilities and reframe dysregulation behaviours from 'naughtiness', therefore avoiding the use of behaviour sanctions.

Sarjit's inclusive values and willingness to work in partnership with colleagues is extremely important in Case Study 2. The professional dialogue was necessary to help her work through her feelings about Jason's behaviour and her worries about what this might say about her professionalism and abilities as a teacher. The case study not only shows a creative and personalised approach to developing tangible support for Jason using a calm down kit but also that relatively straightforward ideas can be transformative for learners. If most people in the class had a calm down kit, Jason would not feel different or singled out – meaning that peer support could also be utilised at appropriate times. The Window of Tolerance theory (Siegel, 1999) is a useful way of thinking about how we function and deal with the day-to-day stresses of life, and is important in this example because it normalises emotions in learning and demonstrates the importance of active and intentional teaching of emotional literacy.

🫴 DEVELOPING EMOTION AND COMMUNICATION FRIENDLY ENVIRONMENTS

One of the benefits of working to develop skills and resources for positive emotional regulation in the classroom is that tools for individual learners often benefit everyone else too. The idea of developing *emotion and communication friendly environments* means that the focus can be on creating the conditions for learners with SLCN to learn alongside their peers and to see challenges and barriers as something that everyone experiences from time to time. It also means that as professionals we are mindful and intentional about the way we bring emotions and learning about them into the classroom space Chang and Taxer (2020). In creating communication friendly classrooms, we would want to think about talking, listening, visual communication and ways for checking understanding (see Chapter 14). To be an emotion - friendly classroom we work to create a classroom space where it feels comfortable to talk about how we feel, to think about how we sit with emotions whether they are positive or negative and building our bodily awareness of the ways that emotions feel.

A strategy for whole class talking about emotions could be developed using an acronym or acrostic. For example, the RULER method developed by Marc Brackett (2019) supports the idea that we must give learners 'permission to feel' and encourage calm and careful reflection on what it means to emotionally regulate. This idea can be adapted to be age specific and could even be devised by a class to give them ownership of their own method. The RULER method considers the following:

R – **Recognition** of emotions in oneself and others

U – **Understanding** the causes and consequences of emotions

L – **Labelling** emotions accurately

E – **Expressing** emotions appropriately

R – **Regulating** emotions effectively

(for more information see: https://www.rulerapproach.org/about/what-is-ruler/ – accessed on 20 January 2025).

Branagan et al.'s (2020) work on emotional regulation offers a holistic framework called 'Language for Behaviour and Emotions' and offers a very comprehensive approach to planning, delivering and evaluating support and interventions for learners with SLCN. It is a highly inclusive resource and can be used by anyone interested in social and emotional wellbeing. It is particular useful for educators because it mirrors a curriculum-based approach and encourages the plan-do-review cycle favoured by SENCos in schools. The LFBE approach works to support learners in the following ways and offers a wide range of resources for professionals to work on aspects such as:

- What to do when things don't make sense (understanding language).
- Saying when you don't understand (comprehension monitoring).
- Understanding words (vocabulary).
- When people don't say what they mean (figurative language).
- Talking about feelings (emotional literacy).
- What's that feeling called? (naming emotions).
- Dealing with feelings (emotional regulation).
- Finding clues and explaining thinking (inference and verbal reasoning).
- The story (narrative).
- Bringing it all together and solving people problems.

(Adapted from Branagan et al., 2020)

CHAPTER SUMMARY

Emotional regulation is a usual and everyday part of being a human in a social setting like a school. It can be tempting to label or categorise learners who find this difficult as 'naughty' or 'challenging'.

- Emotional regulation is important for all learners and will enhance the learning and participation of everyone.
- The role of professionals for supporting positive emotional regulation as one that is important (and often creative).
- An inclusive mindset, where differentiating our work for social and emotional wellbeing is regarded as the same as modifying a mathematics or geography lesson.
- Recognising that learners who need support with emotional dysregulation not as failing, but rather as children and young people who are learning to be in and of the world of the classroom.

As outlined in this chapter, practitioners do need to be able to develop and differentiate their approaches to supporting learners with SCLN. Emotional regulation is not only about individuals in educational settings as they learn in classrooms in a school building, but also cultures and relationships. Working intentionally on the skills and practices of effective emotional regulation can offer some incredibly creative opportunities for professionals to work in partnership – bringing together the expertise of SaLTs and education professionals collaborating for the best outcomes for learners and their families.

Further reading/resources

Branagan, A, Cross, M and Parsons, S (2020) *Language for Behaviour and Emotions: A Practical Guide to Working with Children and Young People*. Routledge.

- This practical, interactive resource is designed to be used by professionals who work with children and young people who have social, emotional and mental health needs and speech, language and communication needs.

RCSLTs factsheet https://www.rcslt.org/wp-content/uploads/media/Project/RCSLT/rcslt-behaviour-a4-factsheet.pdf

- A useful briefing paper from RCSLT that outlines the links between behaviour and communication and gives wider context and definitions of key terminology.

https://library.sheffieldchildrens.nhs.uk/supporting-emotional-regulation-in-early-years/

- This is an example of an NHS Sheffield factsheet that outlines tools for early years settings and outlines the Zones of Regulation approach in an accessible way for busy professionals (see also Chapter 14).

References

Binns, A V, Hutchinson, L R, and Cardy, J O (2019) The speech-language pathologist's role in supporting the development of self-regulation: A review and tutorial. *Journal of Communication Disorders*. March–April; 78:1–17, https://doi.org/10.1016/j.jcomdis.2018.12.005

Brackett, M (2019) *Permission to Feel: Unlock the Power of Emotions to Help Yourself and Your Children Thrive*. New York: Quercus.

Burden, J (2017) *Understanding and supporting children with emotional regulation difficulties*, SENDSupported: embracing difference. Available at: https://www.sendsupported.com/wp-content/uploads/2018/07/emotional-regulation.pdf (accessed 24 February 2025).

Chang, M L and Taxer, J (2020) Teacher emotion regulation strategies in response to classroom misbehavior. *Teachers and Teaching*, 27(5):353–369, https://doi.org/10.1080/13540602.2020.1740198

DfES (2010) Social and emotional aspects of learning (SEAL) programme in secondary schools: national evaluation. Available at: https://www.gov.uk/government/publications/social-and-emotional-aspects-of-learning-seal-programme-in-secondary-schools-national-evaluation (accessed 20 February 2025).

Ecclestone, K and Hayes, D (2009) *The Dangerous Rise of Therapeutic Education*. London: Routledge.

Hobson, H, Brewer, R, Catmur, C, and Bird, G (2019) The role of language in Alexithymia: Moving towards a multiroute model of Alexithymia. *Emotion Review*, 11(3): 247–261, https://doi.org/10.1177/1754073919838528

Jagoe, C and Walsh, I P (eds) (2020) *Communication and Mental Health Disorders: Developing Theory, Growing Practice*. Havant: J and R Press Limited.

Lancastle, D, Davies, N H, Gait, S, Gray, A, John, B, Jones, A, Kunorubwe, T, Molina, J, Roderique-Davies, G, and Tyson, P (2024) A systematic review of interventions aimed at improving emotional regulation in children, adolescents, and adults. *Journal of Behavioral and Cognitive Therapy*, 34(3): 100505, https://doi.org/10.1016/j.jbct.2024.100505

Mayer, R E (2020) Searching for the role of emotions in e-learning. *Learning and Instruction*, 70:101213, https://doi.org/10.1016/j.learninstruc.2019.05.010

NHS (2023) *Mental Health of Children and Young People in England, 2023 - wave 4 follow up to the 2017 survey*. Available at: https://digital.nhs.uk/data-and-information/publications/statistical/mental-health-of-children-and-young-people-in-england/2023-wave-4-follow-up (accessed 24 February 2025).

Oftsed (2024) School inspection handbook. Available at https://www.gov.uk/government/publications/school-inspection-handbook-eif/school-inspection-handbook-for-september-2023

Ripley, K and Yuill, N (2005) Patterns of language impairment and behaviour in boys excluded from school. *British Journal of Educational Psychology*, 75(1): 37–50.

Siegel, D J (1999) *The developing mind*. New York: Guildford.

Steiner, C (1997) *Achieving Emotional Literacy*. New York: Avon.

Weare, K (2013) *Promoting Mental, Emotional and Social Health: A Whole School Approach*. London: Routledge.

Wren, Y, Pagnamenta, E, Orchard, F, Peters, T J, Emond, A, Northstone, K, Miller, L L, and Roulstone, S (2023) Social, emotional and behavioural difficulties associated with persistent speech disorder in children: A prospective population study. *JCPP Advances*, 3(1): e12126. https://doi.org/10.1002/jcv2.12126

5 Multilingualism: Growing up with more than one language

Aydan Suphi

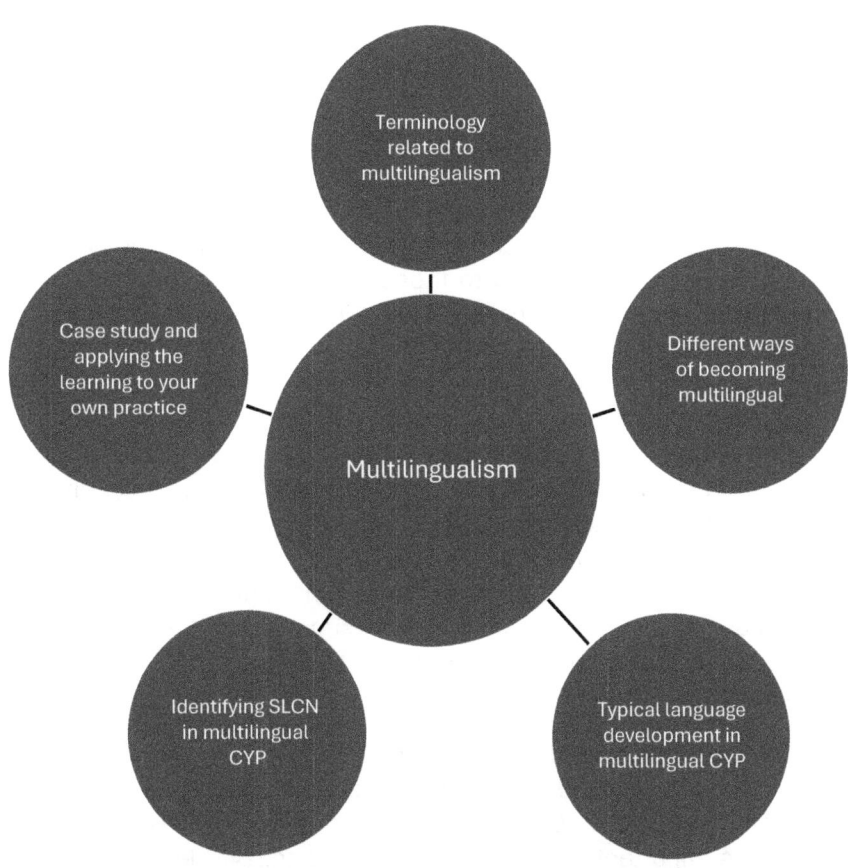

DOI: 10.4324/9781041054986-7

> **CHAPTER OBJECTIVES**
>
> Growing up with more than one language does not cause speech and language difficulties. However, it is important to consider all the languages a child uses when thinking about their speech, language and communication needs. This chapter:
>
> - introduces terminology related to growing up with more than one language;
> - presents the different ways in which children may come to be multilingual;
> - explains typical language development in children and young people (CYP) who are multilingual;
> - discusses challenges and recommendations for identifying speech, language and communication needs in multilingual CYP;
> - considers a case study of a child growing up multilingually and provides critical questions to enable you to apply the learning to your own practice.

Introduction

A variety of terms have been used to describe children who grow up with more than one language. *Bilingual* or *dual language learner* can be used for those who hear, see or learn two languages, and *multilingual* refers to those who know and use more than two languages. However, the terms are sometimes used interchangeably. For simplicity, in this book, we will use *multilingual* to refer to CYP who use two or more languages and monolingual for those who are exposed to only one. Where children start their early years or school setting having had little previous exposure to English, they are typically referred to as having English as an additional language (EAL) (Rutgers et al., 2024). An alternative term, *emergent multilingual (EM)* acknowledges the importance of children continuing to develop their heritage language/s in addition to English (Alanís et al., 2021). Therefore, EM will be used in preference to EAL throughout this book. We will refer to English as the dominant societal language here, while acknowledging that for some parts of the UK, there may be an alternative societal language such as Welsh, Irish or Gaelic. The term 'heritage language' (HL) will be used to refer to the language spoken at home, where it is different from the dominant societal language.

Although the full extent of multilingualism in the UK is not known, the Department for Education (2024) reported that 20.8% of school pupils are EMs. Numbers for nursery-aged children were higher, at 30.7%. Given the large number of CYP who are likely to start school as EMs, it is important to consider how their language development can be supported. Language, culture and identity are intrinsically related, therefore in addressing multilingualism we also must consider the CYP's ethnic and/or religious background and identity. Children learn language within the context of their families and wider communities. It is not only verbal and written language that can differ across cultures, but also gestures, interaction styles and rules of etiquette. CYP who are emerging multilinguals may be growing up with more than one culture that influences their communication.

🏁 STARTING POINTS

- How did you come to learn English, or other languages you know?
- How do the languages you use relate to your cultural identity?
- How have you communicated with CYP who may not yet speak much English?
- How are different cultures and languages celebrated within your place of work?

How do children come to be multilingual?

The circumstances in which CYP come to learn two or more languages may differ between individuals. Yip (2013) and Li (2013) distinguish between two types of multilingual language development:

- Simultaneous language acquisition
- Sequential language acquisition

These will be addressed in turn, giving examples of the contexts in which CYP may be exposed to languages simultaneously and sequentially.

Simultaneous language acquisition

Simultaneous language acquisition refers to children being regularly exposed to two (or more languages) from birth, or before reaching school age (Li, 2013). Children would typically be using both languages regularly during their early childhood (Yip, 2013) and may be exposed to different language through their main caregivers, the wider family and community, preschool settings and media. Table 5.1 shows examples of how children may be exposed to a range of languages in early childhood.

Table 5.1: Examples of language exposure in simultaneous language acquisition

Child	Language A	Language B	Language C
Adem	Mother and her birth family speak their HL, Hungarian, with Adem.	Father and his birth family speak Turkish with Adem. They often watch Turkish TV programmes together.	Mother and Father are proficient in English and speak English together. Adem attends an English-speaking preschool.

Table 5.1 *(Continued)*

Child	Language A	Language B	Language C
Malika	Mother and father speak Somali with each other and their children.	Malika's older sisters learnt English at school and often use it at home. They watch English TV programmes.	The family are Muslim and Arabic prayers are recited regularly in the home.
Holly	Mother is deaf and uses British Sign Language (BSL) with Holly, and with friends and family who know BSL.	Maternal grandmother has hearing and uses English with Holly. Holly attends an English-speaking preschool.	
Ryan	Mother speaks her HL, English, with Ryan.	Father speaks English and Welsh with Ryan. Ryan attends a Welsh language preschool.	

Patterns of language use in a family can be complex. Family members may be multilingual, or parents, siblings or grandparents may speak different languages or vary in their proficiency of each other's main language. In some families, both (or all) languages are used by the whole family. The languages used at any one time may depend on who else is present or on the context. Primary carers may use their HL for nurturing activities, preparing food, for example, and English for talking about educational topics. The family may use their HL at home but change to English when friends or neighbours visit. Alternatively, they may move between English and their HL throughout their conversations (this will be addressed further under the section headed: code-switching). Simultaneous language learners will often start their educational setting with some knowledge of English as well as their HL.

Sequential language acquisition

Sequential language acquisition refers to learning an additional language after preschool age. The lack of agreement amongst authors of a definitive age after which sequential acquisition can be said to occur can make it difficult to distinguish between the two types of language acquisition in young multilinguals (Ortega, 2019; Paradis et al. 2021). A child of three years, who has been exposed only to their HL until they start nursery, for example, could be acquiring language either simultaneously or sequentially, because they are still at preschool age. A clearer example of sequential language acquisition is where a school-age child has recently migrated to the UK with their family, or in the case of older children, sometimes as an unaccompanied asylum seeker. The CYP is likely to be proficient in their HL/s and may have acquired an additional language during their time at a refugee camp in Turkey or Greece for example. They may then learn English sequentially at school.

> **? CRITICAL QUESTIONS**
> - Thinking of CYP you have worked with, would you describe their language acquisition as simultaneous, sequential or a combination of the two?
> - How does their pattern of exposure to different languages compare to the examples in Table 5.1?
> - How much do you know about how they learnt their non-English languages, and the contexts in which they are used in the family?
> - How could you find out this information and what are the possible challenges in doing so?

It is important to understand the pattern of language development in multilinguals to be able to distinguish between those who are developing typically and those who may need additional support with their overall language development. In the following sections we will address what to expect in a child growing up with more than one language.

Language development in multilingual CYP

A key question that concerns educators and speech and language therapists is how multilingual children's language develops compared to that of monolingual children. Few multilinguals are equally competent in all their languages; languages may develop at different rates and the relative competence in each may change over a lifetime (Paradis et al. 2021). Competence in each language depends on a child's age and how frequently they are exposed to the language. Once children start school, they are likely to hear English more frequently and their HL less often. This could result in their English developing more rapidly than their HL (Paradis et al., 2021).

Several research studies have examined vocabulary development in multilingual children. Findings suggest that children learn vocabulary in particular contexts. Therefore, words relating to concepts covered in the school curriculum such as shapes, the planets, the living world, are more likely to be learnt in English, whereas words relevant to home life may be learnt in the HL. By the age of three, sequential multilingual children will typically have acquired words in both languages for some concepts for example 'car' and '*araba*' (Turkish for car); 'dirty' and '*kirli*' (Turkish for dirty). Some languages have a similar sounding word for the same concept, such as 'here' (English) and '*hier*' (German). These are known as cognates. Compared to words that sound very different in each language, for example 'cup' and '*tasse*' (cup in German), cognates are more likely to be learnt in both languages (Paradis et al., 2021).

A typically developing child EM who has not been exposed to English before may at first try to use their HL at school, but if there is no one who understands that language, they will quickly stop using it (Tabors et al., 2008). Having a member of staff or another child who speaks their HL may help them to settle into school life. Older children are sometimes self-conscious about using their HL at school and may avoid doing so. It is important to be encouraging and validating of their multilingual ability and identity (see guidance in Table 5.2. below). In the early stages of being in a second-language environment, CYP may go through what has been termed the 'silent period' where they communicate only through non-verbal means, such as pointing and nodding. This varies across EMs with some having no silent period and others being silent from a few weeks to several months. After this time, EMs typically start using single words or short phrases in English and then go on to use a wider range of words and construct longer sentences. The length of time it takes for EMs to reach functional use of English can vary but typically, they will have acquired some level of competence in their first year of attending (an English-speaking) school.

Patterns of development can be different for sequential learners of English than for simultaneous multilinguals or monolingual English speakers. The phonology (sound system) of all languages is different and CYP may produce consonants or vowels differently to monolingual speakers. An example is the sound 'W' which does not exist in languages such as Turkish. Turkish-English EMs therefore commonly use 'V' instead of 'W' when speaking English. Similarly, sound blends such as 'sp' in 'spade' may be changed by inserting a vowel so that it sounds like 'sapade'. These are multilingual variations of English and should not be confused with speech sound disorders, which will be covered in Chapter 6.

Table 5.2 *Guidance for supporting multilingual learners*

- Find out as much as you can about the CYP's patterns of language use, for example, where and when each language is used and when it was learnt.
- Celebrate and reinforce the CYP's multilingualism as a strength, and an important part of their identity.
- Reassure and encourage parents to continue to use their HL with their child at home.
- When CYP start school with little or no functional use of English, expect that they may take some time to start to speak.
- Use short simple language to give information and use visuals such as gesture and pointing to pictures or symbols to help the CYP to understand.
- For older CYP, simple written instructions may be easier to understand than spoken information.
- Encourage the CYP to communicate in any way they can or feel comfortable. This includes speaking in their HL if there are other students or members of staff who can interpret, or by using gestures.
- Find out from parents if there are any concerns about the CYP's speech and language development in their HL/s, for example, whether they are understanding and using speech and language in a similar way to other children the same age.
- Where there are concerns about the CYP's language development, assessment should be carried out in all their languages to gain an accurate picture of their abilities and needs.

Grammatical differences can also be seen in the English of EMs. Pronouns (e.g. he, she), irregular forms of past tense (e.g. came; ran) or plurals (e.g. children; sheep) can be problematic. Learning grammar may not be a linear process, with EMs using the standard English form at times and not at others (Paradis et al. 2021). Again, this is not indicative of a language disorder that requires intervention, unless there are concerns about the child's grammatical development across all their languages.

Code-switching

Code-switching is a typical behaviour in multilinguals. This refers to using both languages within a conversation. Speakers may change language between utterances, between or within sentences or even within words. An example of a within-word code-switch is where the root of the word is in one language and the marker for plurals or tenses in another as demonstrated below:

'dinosaur*lar*' (dinosaurs)

The Turkish suffix *lar*, indicating a plural, is added to the English word dinosaur.

Contrary to popular misconception, code-switching does not necessarily indicate a lack of proficiency in one or both languages. Typically, developing multilinguals usually code-switch only when talking with others who understand both languages. The code-switch can serve many different purposes, for example, demonstrating belonging to a multilingual community. Code-switching within a conversation may indicate a change of topic, it may be used to quote what others have said or may occur because there is a better way of expressing the idea in one language compared to the other.

Assessing language development in multilingual children

When considering whether a child's language is developing typically, it is important to consider all their languages. This is relevant for any assessments of language carried out across age groups. Assessing in only one language can put multilingual children at a disadvantage. An example of this is where a child's vocabulary is assessed in English only. In comparison with monolingual English speakers, multilingual CYP's vocabulary may appear more limited. However, when their whole vocabulary is considered, (counting any words they know in both languages once only) multilingual CYP have been found to have vocabularies equivalent to, or larger than that of monolingual CYP of the same age and socio-economic background.

Multilingual CYP can also be disadvantaged by the resources used to assess their language ability. Some assessment tools have been designed for and standardised on monolingual English-speaking CYP, resulting in inaccurate or invalid results when used with multilinguals. To limit bias in assessment it is also important to consider whether the resources used (such as pictures or words assessed) are culturally appropriate for, and representative of CYP from ethnic minority families. Language is culturally linked, and children are more likely to know words relating to foods, items and events relevant to their daily lives. Pictures depicting people who look and dress differently to their family, or scenarios that are outside a child's experience may be more difficult for them to relate to and talk about. Expectations regarding how a child communicates may also differ across cultures. In British schools, initiating a conversation with an adult may be seen as desirable and indicative of good communication development. However, in other cultures this may not be considered appropriate behaviour for a child, therefore it is important to try to understand family expectations of typical and appropriate communication.

Multilingualism does not cause speech and language disorders. However, as for monolingual children, some multilinguals will experience difficulties with their speech and language development. Children with SLCN such as developmental language disorder, phonological difficulties or any of the other difficulties covered in this book will experience it across all their languages. Multilingual children are at risk of being over-identified as having SLCN if they are only assessed in English. Conversely, SLCN can be missed in multilingual CYP if it is assumed that any differences in communication are due to them having had insufficient exposure to English. Appropriate assessment should include discussion with the child's family regarding the languages spoken at home, and their views on their child's speech and language development, for example, compared to other children in the family. Children who are EM and do not have SLCN or other difficulties will typically show progress in learning to understand and use English words over time and will be able to communicate well in their HL.

Supporting the development of multilingual children

It is now widely recognised that it is beneficial for parents to speak with their child in the language/s most natural to them (usually their HL/s). This is likely to provide children with rich models of language as well as supporting their sense of cultural belonging. Cultural traditions, stories and songs are often passed to younger generations through language (Grosjean, 2024). By learning the HL/s of the family, a child can communicate with members of the wider family and their cultural community. However, there are many factors that may influence parents' decision about which language/s to use with their child. These include the political context, advice given by professionals and parents' varying beliefs about multilingualism. Languages differ in their perceived or actual status within a country. Languages of communities who are minoritised (and therefore hold less power in society) have lower status than the societal language. Some parents may choose to speak English with their child, rather than their HL, because they believe this to be necessary for their child's academic and future success. In some cases, parents have also been inappropriately advised by health and education professionals to use only English with their child at home, particularly where the child has additional needs.

In a country where monolingualism has historically largely been seen as the norm, active celebration of multilingualism may support parents to make a more informed choice about the languages they use with their children. As educators we can celebrate the beauty of multilingualism and the way CYP skilfully navigate between their languages. Research evidence has shown that multilingualism does not cause SLCN (Peña, 2016). Despite assumptions that learning two languages increases pressure on children with SLCN, research findings suggest that children with additional needs, raised multilingually, can learn to communicate just as well or even better than those raised with one language. Emerging evidence suggests that multilingualism can benefit both social and cognitive development. Although the findings have not been definitive, potential cognitive advantages include enhanced attention control, impulse inhibition and flexible thought (Antoniou, 2019).

SPOTLIGHT ON CURRENT DEBATES ABOUT MULTILINGUALISM

Traditionally monolingualism and multilingualism have been labelled as distinct categories. However, more recently it has been proposed that language use would be more accurately described as a continuum with monolingualism at one end and multilingualism at the other. The dynamic process of language learning means that an individual can move along the continuum from monolingual towards multilingual over time (Ortega 2019).

There have also been ongoing debates about the distinction between language and dialect. Traditionally, *language* has been used to refer to the formal, 'standard' version of English as used by the dominant elite, for example, with variations referred to as *dialects* (Flores and Schissel, 2014). This has been challenged as problematic for the following reasons. Caribbean creoles such as Jamaican Patois have often been considered as a dialect of standard English. This has resulted in children from African-Caribbean backgrounds being corrected for not speaking 'White Mainstream English' (Baker-Bell, 2020 p. 9). In comparison with those starting school speaking a different *language* to English, it has been argued that children speaking a non-standard *dialect* of English are disadvantaged. Not only is their language seen as deficient (compared to standard academic English), but they also miss out on support given to children who are considered EMs.

A perhaps more radical debate is the question of whether individual languages really exist. Wei and Garćia (2022) suggest that rather than focusing on individual languages such as English and Arabic as monolingual speakers use them, we should consider a multilingual learner's languages in combination. A learner who is exposed to English and Arabic may use either, both or combine the two. They refer to this as *translanguaging*. While the idea of complete fluidity between languages may be a far stretch for some, the importance of considering the learner's full repertoire of languages when assessing their communication skills is important and valid.

CASE STUDY

Siân is a nursery teacher in a multicultural urban area

We have a lot of children who have not been exposed to much English before they start nursery, for example, most of them can say 'hello' in English, but that might be all. We use a total communication approach with our children with SEND and some of this helps our EM children too. We have picture symbols that we carry on lanyards, and this helps the children understand what we mean if they don't know English. We find Makaton signs are more helpful for them though when they want to tell us something. We also have songs for different activities and the EM children often start to join in with words or actions. I always say that the additional resources we have in class to support children with additional needs never harm the rest of the children, it only enhances their learning. We often have Mr Tumble on while the children are getting their coats, and it means that all the children learn about Makaton signs and can use them with each other.

I always encourage parents to speak their HL with their children. Sometimes parents will proudly tell you that they are speaking English with their child and learning with them, but we find that the child then misses out on having conversations in their HL and this can mean that they find it difficult to express themselves in either their HL or English. The Book Trust has previously given us books to send home with children. Now, they are providing books in the children's HLs too, so we can support parents with shared book reading at home. The children in my class speak ten different languages and we have been able to get books in all their languages, including Punjabi, Urdu, Bengali, Kurdish and Romanian. This will hopefully encourage parents to continue to have conversations with their children in their HLs, while we support them with English at nursery (Table 5.3).

⑦ Critical questions

- What visual strategies do you use, or could you adopt to support your EM learners?
- What could you do in your setting to promote the use of HLs at home?
- How would you respond to parents telling you that they are speaking English with their child, in preference to their HL/s?

 Table 5.3 Indicators that multilingual CYP require assessment of their speech, language and communication needs

CYP may require assessment of their speech and language skills if:
• Parents report concerns about the CYP's speech and language in the HL
• Parents are unable to understand what the child is saying after the age of three

(Continued)

Table 5.3 (Continued)

• The CYP is unable to follow instructions or express themselves in the language they know best
• Parents report that the CYP is not using speech and language in the same way as other children in the family at the same age
• Where there has been direct teaching of vocabulary or grammar in English, the CYP finds it difficult to retain what has been taught
• The CYP is showing distress or frustration about not being able to communicate. This may manifest as unwelcome behaviours, emotional outbursts or withdrawal

CHAPTER SUMMARY

A large proportion of CYP grow up multilingually. Some will be exposed to more than one language simultaneously in their early years, while others will learn one language before acquiring another (sequential language learning). Multilingual CYP may have different levels of competence in each of their languages, depending on how frequently and where they are exposed to them. When considering their overall language competence, their abilities across all their languages should be considered. Comparing their ability in one language only (such as English) to that of monolingual children may result in false identification of SLCN. HLs are an important part of a child or young person's identity and allowing their learning of them allows for communication with community and family members. Growing up with more than one language should be encouraged and celebrated. Multilingualism does not cause SLCN but just as for monolinguals, some multilingual CYP will present with SLCN.

Further reading/resources

Q-BEX is an online questionnaire which can be used with parents of multilingual children to find out about their language exposure in different languages. As it is designed for research purposes, the questionnaire is quite detailed but some of the questions can be useful for gathering information about how different languages are used in the child's life. Available at: www.q-bex.org

Tiny Happy People is a BBC website with short videos and advice aimed at supporting families with their preschool children's language development. There is a useful section on guidance on raising children multilingually. Available at: https://www.bbc.co.uk/tiny-happy-people/bilingual

References

Alanís, I, Arreguín, M G, and Salinaz-González, I (2021) *The Essentials: Dual Language Learners in Diverse Environments in Preschool and Kindergarten*. La Vergne: National association for the education of young children.

Antoniou, M (2019) The advantages of bilingualism debate. *Annual Review of Linguistics*, 5: 395–415.

Baker-Bell, A (2020) Dismantling anti-black linguistic racism in English language arts classrooms: Toward an anti-racist black language pedagogy. *Theory into Practice*, 59(1): 8–21.

Department for Education (2024) *Schools, pupils and their characteristics: Academic year 2023/24*. [online] Available at: https://explore-education-statistics.service.gov.uk/find-statistics.school-pupils-and-their-characteristics (Accessed 13 March 2025).

Flores, N and Schissel, J L (2014) Dynamic bilingualism as the norm: Envisioning a heteroglossic approach to standards-based reform. *TESOL Quarterly*, 48(3): 454–479.

Grosjean, F (2024) *On Bilinguals and Bilingualism*. Cambridge: Cambridge University Press.

Li, P (2013) Successive language acquisition. In: Grosjean, F and Li, P (Eds) *The psycholinguistics of bilingualism*. Chichester: Wiley-Blackwell pp. 145–167.

Ortega, L (2019) The study of heritage language development from a bilingualism and social justice perspective. *Language Learning* 70 (S1): 15–53.

Paradis, J, Genesee, F and Crago, M B (2021) *Dual language development and disorders: A handbook on bilingualism and second language learning*. 3rd edition. Baltimore: Paul H. Brookes Publishing.

Peña, E D (2016) Supporting the home language of children with developmental disabilities: From knowing to doing. *Journal of Communication Disorders*, 63: 85–92.

Rutgers, D, Evans, M, Fisher, L, Forbes, K, Gayton, A, and Liu, Y (2024) Multilingualism, Multilingual identity and academic attainment: Evidence from secondary schools in England. *Journal of Language, Identity and Education*, 23(2): 210–227.

Tabors, P, Snow, C E, and Paez, M (2008) *One Child, Two Languages: A Guide for Early Childhood Educators of Children Learning English as a Second Language*. 2nd ed. Baltimore: Brookes Publishing.

Wei, L and Garćia, O (2022) Not a first language but one repertoire: Translanguaging as a decolonising project. *RELC Journal*, 53(2): 313–324.

Yip, V (2013) Simultaneous language acquisition. In: Grosjean, F and Li, P (Eds) *The psycholinguistics of bilingualism*. Chichester: Wiley-Blackwell pp. 121–144.

SECTION II KEY SPEECH, LANGUAGE, AND COMMUNICATION AREAS

6 Speech

Charlie Ayling and Lorraine Bamblett

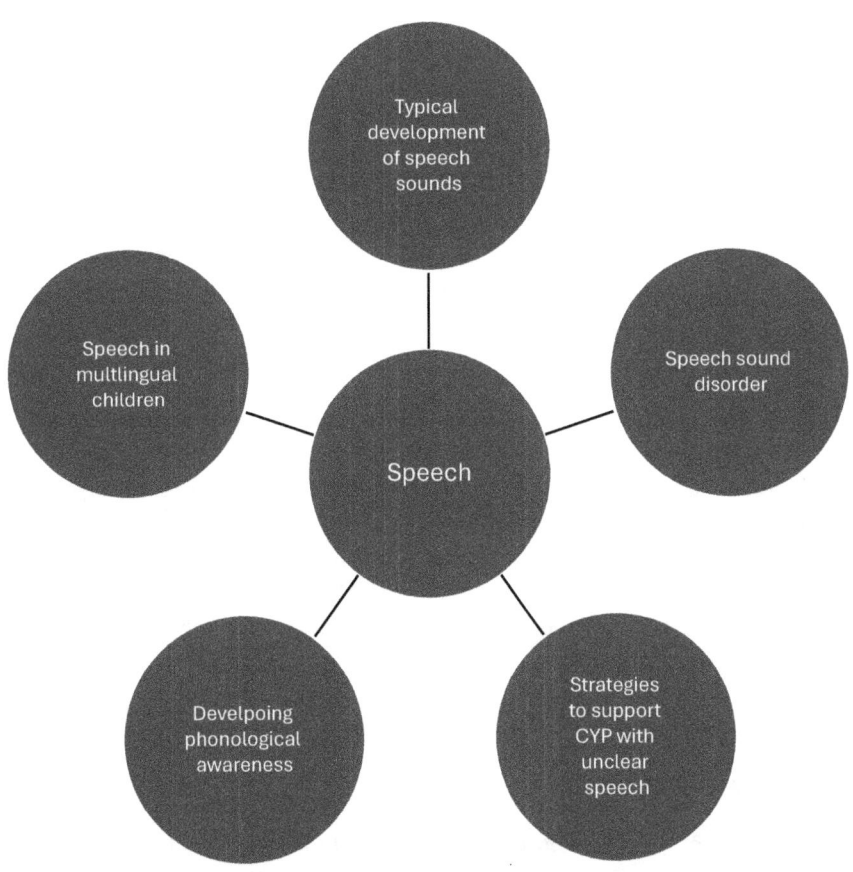

DOI: 10.4324/9781041054986-9

CHAPTER OBJECTIVES

This chapter discusses speech sound development and its impact on language, learning and literacy skills. The chapter:

- introduces key terminology;
- describes typical and atypical development of speech sounds, with information about when to refer to speech and language therapy for support;
- discusses links between speech sound development and outcomes for learning, literacy, language and wellbeing;
- identifies strategies and interventions to develop children and young people's (CYP) speech and support them in the classroom.

Introduction

Speech refers to the ability to pronounce individual sounds (vowels and consonants) and use them in words. This skill typically develops from an early age when children start to make sounds (babbling) to around seven years when most sounds should be acquired. Difficulties with pronunciation of speech sounds can be referred to as Speech Sound Disorder (SSD) which impact a child's ability to make themselves understood and to express their thoughts, needs and ideas. SSDs can impact not only a child's emotional and social wellbeing but also their educational outcomes, with robustly evidenced links between SSD and difficulties with vocabulary, reading and spelling (Wren et al., 2021).

Pupils with SSD tend to have associated difficulties with phonological awareness (awareness of how sounds fit together to make words) which affects their ability to identify, segment and blend phonemes (single consonants and vowels) integral to phonics instruction. Early support with phonological awareness is crucial and can be integrated into classroom practice to develop CYP's readiness for literacy instruction (see Chapter 8 for more information on this). It is important for educators to have an awareness of speech sound development to identify when onward referral to speech and language therapy services may be required.

STARTING POINTS

- What kind of activities might a child with unclear speech find difficult in the classroom?
- What does this mean for how you check their understanding, or assess their knowledge verbally?
- How can teaching staff support a child experiencing unclear speech with their participation in class?

Typical development of speech sounds

Children develop speech sounds gradually and the time it takes to do so can vary, with some naturally taking longer than others. The age and order of speech sounds developed is different across languages. Children who speak more than one language are not at higher risk for difficulties with speech sounds but will develop the sounds they need for all languages at different rates depending on the amount of exposure they have to each language. Posters showing the typical development of consonant sounds in English are included in the key resources at the end of the chapter (Table 6.1).

Table 6.1 The age at which 90% of children develop consonant sounds in English (McLeod and Crowe, 2018:1558)

Age	Consonant sounds acquired
2 years	p
3 years	b
	t
	d
	c/k
	g
	m
	n
	f
	h
	y
	w
4 years	v
	s
	z
	sh
	ch
	j
	l
5 years	th
	r

Due to this developmental progression, the speech of younger children will sound different to adult speech, but this is not always a cause for concern, depending on their age and which sounds they are having difficulty with. Generally, most people should be able to understand what a child is saying in their main language by the time they are four years old, even though it is likely they still have some sounds that are developing (e.g. 'th' and 'r' in English-speaking children).

As children do not have all the required speech sounds from the beginning, there are types of errors (or error patterns) that children tend to make at certain ages as they simplify words (Bamblett et al., forthcoming). Table 6.2 shows the main error patterns found in typical development of English, with examples of how words may sound and the age that children usually stop making these errors.

Table 6.2 *Typical speech error patterns (Dodd, Holm, Hua and Crosbie, 2003)*

Speech error type	Description and examples	Typical age
Final consonant deletion	Deleting (not saying) the final consonant on a word. Cat – 'ca' Dog – 'do'	Up to age 2
Voicing	Replacing quiet (voiceless) speech sounds with louder (voiced) ones. This relates to vibration of the vocal cords. 'p' said as 'b' (pig – 'big') 't' said as 'd' (toy = 'doy')	Up to age 3
Stopping	Replacing long fricative sounds (f, v, s, z, sh) with short plosive sounds (p, b, t, d, c/k, g). Sun – 'dun' Four – 'boor' or 'door'	Up to age 3½
Weak syllable deletion	Deleting (not saying) 1 or more syllables in a word. Elephant – 'efant' (3 syllables reduced to 2) Pushing – 'pu' (2 syllables reduced to 1)	Up to age 4
Fronting	Replacing sounds made at the back of the mouth (c/k, g) with sounds made at the front of the mouth (t, d). Car – 'tar' Gate – 'date'	Up to age 4
Cluster reduction (2 consonants together)	Reducing a 2-element consonant cluster (2 consonant sounds together like cl, fl, br, pr, sp, st, etc.) down to 1 sound. Spider – 'pider' or 'bider' Blue – 'boo'	Up to age 4

Table 6.2 (Continued)

Speech error type	Description and examples	Typical age
Cluster reduction (3 consonants together)	Reducing a 3-element consonant cluster (3 consonant sounds together like spr, scr, str etc) down to one sound. Strawberry – 'sawberry' or 'tawberry'	Up to age 5
Deaffrication	Difficulty saying 'ch' and 'j' sounds, may be replaced with a fricative sound like 's' or 'sh' or a plosive sound 't' or 'd'. Bridge – 'bridz' or 'briss' Chair – 'tear' or 'share'	Up to age 5
Gliding	Replacing 'l' and 'r' sounds with 'w' and/or 'y'. Red – 'wed' Lock – 'yock'	Up to age 6

NB children can use different sounds to the ones used in these examples.

Speech Sound Disorder

Speech Sound Disorder (SSD) is an umbrella term used to cover a range of difficulties that some children have with their speech (pronunciation of sounds in words) over and above the typical developmental sequence. You may have heard of other terms being used to describe these difficulties, including speech delay, speech impairment, articulation difficulty and verbal dyspraxia.

Children with SSD have patterns of errors in their speech that make it difficult to understand what they are saying. They might remove (or add) a sound in a word (e.g. saying 'ca' instead of cat), or they might replace sounds they cannot say with easier sounds (e.g. using an earlier developing sound like 't' in place of a later developing sound like 'ch', saying 'tip' instead of chip). As described above, some of these error patterns typically occur naturally in developing young children as they learn to use more complex speech sounds. However, some children continue to show these error patterns as they get older (often labelled as speech delay), and some children have error patterns that are not typically seen in younger children (often labelled as speech disorder). Around 12 in every 100 children have SSD, and half of them have associated language difficulties (RCSLT, 2024), see Chapter 7 for more information on language.

SSDs can be categorised based on the nature of the difficulty into articulation (including motor speech) and phonology.

- Articulation relates to making movements required for speech, meaning that the child cannot copy a sound or produces a distorted version (e.g. interdental lisp, where a child puts their tongue between their teeth when saying 's' making it sound like 'th'). Most children with articulation disorders have no associated difficulties with movement in general, but some are related to cleft lip and palate or other disabilities like cerebral palsy.

- Motor speech disorders, including Childhood Apraxia of Speech and Childhood Dysarthria, are also related to making and coordinating the required movements for speech but tend to have a more significant and long-term impact. Children with motor speech disorders often have a limited range of sounds that they can say correctly in words and might say words differently each time they attempt them, meaning that these children are unintelligible even to close family members.

- Phonology relates to the storage of words in a person's brain. CYP may be able to say a sound correctly on its own but make errors with the sound in words because they have stored an incorrect/errored version of the word. For example, some children use 't' in place of 'c/k' at an early age because they have not yet developed 'c/k' and will say 'tat' in place of 'cat'. This then becomes stored in their brain after saying it many times and so even when they are older and can say the 'c/k' sound accurately they still make this error.

Children with SSD need support from speech and language therapists to identify the cause of the difficulty and provide appropriate recommendations. This might include listening to the difference between sounds they make errors with, teaching them how to say a new sound or practising sounds within words. Changing the way words are stored in a CYP's brain is a difficult process, they need to say the new correct version of a word many times before a strong connection is made and they can retrieve this version when they speak in conversation. This means that even when a child can say a word correctly with support, they might not be doing so in their natural communication right away and are not being 'lazy' when they make mistakes.

Table 6.3 shows error patterns that are not typically found in development and are considered indicators of a disorder (in English).

Table 6.3 Atypical speech error patterns

Speech error type	Description and examples
Backing	Replacing sounds made at the front of the mouth (p, b, t, d, f, s) with sounds made at the back (c/k, g). Sock – 'gock' Teddy – 'keggy'
Affrication	Replacing short plosive sounds (p, b, t, d, c/k, g) with long fricative sounds (f, s, sh, ch). Dog – 'zog' Teeth – 'cheef'
Initial consonant deletion	Removing (not saying) the first consonant in a word, meaning that the word starts with a vowel sound. This applies only to single consonants (e.g. 't') rather than consonant clusters (e.g. 'tr'). Bee – 'ee' Game – 'ame'

Table 6.3 (Continued)

Speech error type	Description and examples
Favourite sound	Replacing lots of sounds with one favoured sound, for example a child may use 'd' in place of 't', 'c/k', 'g', 'f', 's', 'sh', etc. Chair, care, stare, fair, tear, share – 'dare'
Nasal emission	Nasal emission (air coming down the nose) which may be heard alongside an 's' sound, or instead of it (you may not hear the 's' at all and just some air escaping down the child's nose).
Inconsistency	Children say the same word in a different way each time they say it and the word sounds very unusual. This does not apply where the child sometimes gets a sound right and sometimes does not as this is most likely to be related to them learning the new sound (e.g. they can say 'car' correctly but not 'cat').

 Children should be referred for SLT assessment where they are:

- over four years old and very difficult to understand;
- regularly using one or more typical speech error types and over six months past the expected age;
- regularly using any of the atypical speech error patterns;
- over three years old and making errors with vowel sounds (a, o, oo, ee, etc.).

 SPOTLIGHT ON EMERGING DEBATES

Speech development in children who speak multiple languages

Around 9% of UK residents do not report English as their main language, according to the 2021 census, and this is increasing year on year. Many CYP are growing up in multilingual homes and although this is not a cause of speech and language difficulties, as education practitioners we need to understand the challenges that identifying and supporting SLCN in multilingual pupils involves. We need to recognise indicators of SSD and ensure that support is put in place so we can avoid inequalities in our practice.

Children develop separate phonological systems for each language that they hear and speak (Holm et al., 1999). This means that they store words and sounds for each language separately and so speech errors can often be different across languages and error patterns can be resolved at different times (Pert, 2023). Therefore, it can be difficult to identify whether a child has SSD, particularly in languages where there is less published information about development of sounds and the error patterns to expect. A slightly slower rate of development of speech sounds in one of a CYP's spoken languages may not indicate a disorder, CYP with SSD will have difficulties across their languages.

We cannot rely on the use of typical developmental milestones to identify SSD in multilingual children as these are based on monolingual children (speaking one language only) and there will be many individual differences relating to the age at which a child started learning each language and the amount of exposure they have to them, as well as the differing phonological make-up of languages that is likely to impact development. This can make it challenging to work out whether a pupil is displaying typical multilingual speech or potential SSD.

If you have concerns about a CYP's speech in English, speak to their family and ask if they also have concerns in their home language/s. If they do, or you are still unsure, refer to speech and language therapy services so that the process of differentiating between typical development and SSD for the individual CYP can be considered further. This should involve working with the pupil's family to gather information about their language use and assessing the pupil's speech in their home language/s. The advice and strategies shared later in this chapter can still be used to support children's speech, whatever language/s they speak.

Supporting children with unclear speech

The main ways you can support pupils with unclear speech in the classroom are:

- Focusing on what the CYP is saying, not how they are saying it. CYP with SSD can be very aware of their difficulties, which impacts on their self-esteem.

- Modelling accurate speech, repeating back the word as it should be said. Do not correct the child, or ask them to repeat, but give them an opportunity to hear the word said accurately (e.g. Child: 'Tup'. Adult: 'Yes, it's a cup'.) NB Adults do this because they want to encourage the child to say the word correctly, but this can cause significant frustration for children who cannot say the sound yet, or those who are not aware that their version of the word sounds different. It is more helpful for the CYP to hear the correct version and see how you move your mouth when you say the sounds.

- Emphasising sounds in your own speech and providing opportunities for them to hear and see key sounds in writing. Draw attention to their tricky sounds when reading stories or during phonics.

- Using cued articulation in phonics. This was developed by the SaLT, Jane Passey in the 1970s and is a set of hand signals for spoken consonants and vowels. It is widely used by SaLTs when working with children with SSD to give them visual clues to help them understand where in the mouth different sounds are made. See Chapter 14 for an example of how these can be used in phonics for all children. We have included links and resources to help you implement cued articulation with your pupils.

- Being mindful of their peer's reactions to their speech, CYP can be judged by others for the way the speak and this can lead to isolation and bullying.
- Using a home-school communication book, or diary, where information can be shared between home and school about key people in the CYP's life and activities they are likely to want to talk to you about in school. Remember that CYP with SSD are not always able to tell their family members about what they have done in school.
- Considering reasonable adjustments – how can the CYP with unclear speech be supported to demonstrate their learning or contribute to classroom discussions? This might include creating opportunities for them to show their learning non-verbally, collecting information about their error patterns so they can engage in phonics/language screening, or requesting support from a familiar adult who is tuned in to their speech and can interpret for them.
- Working towards their speech targets little and often across the week; regular practice leads to faster progress and reduces negative outcomes.

If you are having difficulty understanding something a CYP is saying, repeat back the part you think you have understood to check it is correct. Ask them to show you or use a gesture to help you understand the rest or offer choices (e.g. 'Is it Lego or trains?').

Developing phonological awareness

Phonological awareness (awareness of sounds in words) is an essential skill for using the correct speech sounds in words, learning vocabulary and developing literacy skills (Stringer, 2019). Phonological awareness starts with larger units, understanding how to split a sentence into words and segmenting or manipulating syllables within words (e.g. tomato 'to-ma-to') (Anthony and Francis, 2005). Pupils then develop the ability to identify phonemes by around five years of age (typically starting with initial and final) with awareness of rhyme coming later. It is typical that a pupil of seven years of age may only just be able to make rhyme judgements or generate rhyming words. CYP can usually identify whether phonemes are the same or different before they can manipulate them and can blend before they can segment. A high percentage of children with SLCN have difficulties with phonological awareness that impact on literacy development.

Stringer (2019) has produced a free to download whole class screening and intervention package designed to be implemented in early years settings, although it is suitable for older children. She advocates for children to develop these fundamental skills, such as syllable segmentation, syllable deletion and initial and final sound substitution before they progress into Reception class. The link to these resources can be found in Further reading/resources.

Working on phonological awareness skills has been proven to impact children's literacy and phonological development whether or not they are at risk of SLCN and/or literacy

CASE STUDY

Nina, SENCo in a mainstream primary school

Hedley, a 6-year-old boy with severe SSD and presenting with traits of ADHD, was an engaging and lively pupil with lots of good ideas. Hedley was often upset because he found it hard to make and sustain friendships. He was regularly singled out as the cause of 'trouble' at lunchtime, and other children would complain about his playground etiquette. Hedley's family were very supportive of school but concerned that his speech was still very unclear despite the involvement of SLT services, and that he was struggling with basic literacy and number skills. Hedley was also quite clumsy and accident-prone.

In order to support Hedley, a number of strategies were put into place.

Seating placement

Hedley disliked being at the front of class but needed to be placed where he could have additional support from a 'floating' class TA. In common with many children with SLCN, he was prone to copying from peers. It was vital that we were able to ensure that he wasn't copying because he hadn't understood or followed instructions, or because the task was not well matched to his level of attainment and proximal next steps. Being near a TA also meant that he had someone to hand that was a familiar listener so she could *interpret any questions* or comments that Hedley had about the learning task.

Learning environment

The classroom was communication friendly, with learning walls to refer to, sign-supported English, visual timetables, a clutter-free environment and well-labelled resources among the strategies employed. Phonics were taught using signs from cued articulation which gave Hedley daily reminders of how to make each speech sound.

Support

The floating TA and teacher were both aware that Hedley would need support to stay on task and to complete any given task and would make sure to check in with him frequently during the session.

Relationships

It was critical for all staff working in the room to develop a good relationship with Hedley, who was quite attention-intensive and could easily develop rejection sensitivity from his formative experiences of being told to wait for help or if he wasn't understood by peers.

This often led to miscommunication and fall-outs with peers. Adults had noticed he was often the centre of arguments on the playground.

Intervention

Hedley's speech sound programme was delivered three times a week as directed by his SLT. He also received daily additional phonics sessions as he was part of the 'bottom 20%' of readers. Elklan-trained staff in school knew to let him finish what he was saying and familiar staff were 'tuned in' to his speech, although it was necessary to ask him to repeat himself or employ signs, drawings and at times pointing to help mediate his speech. Incorrect speech productions were modelled back correctly so Hedley heard the correct way of saying words.

Social support

Hedley took part in Time To Talk, and time was taken daily to talk through any incidents on the playground in an unofficial 'circle of friends' approach so that he was able to voice his perspective as well as hear his peer's perspective. The disagreements were often either around Hedley not understanding his peer's intentions or his peer not understanding what Hedley was asking of him because of his SSD. He was also quite physical, a trait seen often in children with SLCN – where physical action is less tiring than trying to understand or express the nuances of language. It was important that his peers were able to begin to understand why he behaved as he did, but also for him to understand how his actions were seen by his peers in order to make choices that enable better relationships between them. Training was also done with lunchtime staff to explain how important validating feelings and listening to children's viewpoints was during playtime altercations.

⑦ Critical questions

- Is the whole child being supported? Hedley's whole experience of education could have been very negative if his social difficulties and impact of his SSD led to constant feelings of rejection.
- What more could we have done for Hedley – are there any supports for his speech sounds that could have been put in place to potentially mitigate the impact on his behaviour?

difficulties, so there is an argument for implementing this as a universal approach. There is a large overlap of children who are at risk of both SSD and literacy difficulties due to an overall impairment in phonological awareness that underpins skills in reading, writing and speech sound development. We know how important these skills are to academic success and employment in later life.

> **CHAPTER SUMMARY**
>
> This chapter introduced readers to typical speech development in English before focusing on speech sound disorders and their impact on wellbeing, language and literacy. We have considered identification of SSD in children who speak multiple languages and provided strategies and resources to support CYP in whatever language/s they speak.

Further reading/resources

- Public information about speech sound disorders from the Royal College of Speech and Language Therapists: https://www.rcslt.org/speech-and-language-therapy/clinical-information/speech-sound-disorders/.

- McLeod and Crowe (2018) Phoneme development in English around the world https://www.csu.edu.au/research/multilingual-speech/speech-acquisition/learning-english-consonants.

- Cued articulation can be used within phonics sessions for all children to support their learning of consonants and vowels. See https://www.soundsforliteracy.com.au/index.html for more information on how you can implement it and how to access online training. For a DVD with cued articulation videos suitable for whiteboards, please see https://www.elklan.co.uk/Shop/Cued_Articulation_DVD.

- For access to the free download of the Newcastle Assessment for Phonological Awareness and the Newcastle Intervention for Phonological Awareness, please see https://research.ncl.ac.uk/phonologicalawareness/assessmentandintervention/downloadthenipaandnapa/ – this also includes commentary on how this highly evidence-based programme can be used in schools across the key stages.

References

Anthony, J L and Francis, D J (2005) Development of phonological awareness. *Current Directions in Psychological Science*, 14(5): 255–259. doi:10.1111/j.0963-7214.2005.00376.x

Bamblett, L, Amer-El-Khedoud, M, Ayling, C and Madigan, B (forthcoming) *Working with Children's Speech Sound Disorders: A Practical Guide for Speech and Language Therapists*. Oxon: Routledge.

Dodd, B, Holm, A, Hua, Z, and Crosbie, S (2003) Phonological development: A normative study of British English-speaking children. *Clinical Linguistics & Phonetics*, 17(8): 617–643. https://doi.org/10.1080/0269920031000111348

Holm, A, Dodd, B, Stow, C, and Pert, S (1999) Identification and differential diagnosis of phonological disorder in bilingual children. *Language Testing*, 16(3): 271–292. 2. https://doi.org/10.1191/026553299674008527

McLeod, S and Crowe, K (2018) Children's consonant acquisition in 27 languages: A cross-linguistic review. *American Journal of Speech-Language Pathology*, 27: 1546–1571. https://doi.org/10.1044/2018_AJSLP-17-0100

Pert, S (2023) *Working with Children Experiencing Speech and Language Disorders in a Bilingual Context. A Home Language Approach*. Abingdon: Routledge.

RCSLT (2024) Speech Sound Disorders Clinical Guidance – accessed from: https://www.rcslt.org/members/clinical-guidance/speech-sound-disorders/speech-sound-disorders-guidance

Stringer, H (2019) *Newcastle Assessment for Phonological Awareness*. 1st edition Newcastle upon Tyne: Newcastle University, School of Education, Communication and Language Sciences.

Wren, Y, Pagnamenta, E, Peters, TJ, Emond, A, Northstone, K, Miller, LL, and Roulstone, S (2021) Educational outcomes associated with persistent speech disorder. *International Journal of Language & Communication Disorders*, 56(2), 299–312. https://doi.org/10.1111/1460-6984.12599

7 Understanding and using language

Lorraine Bamblett and Natacha Capener

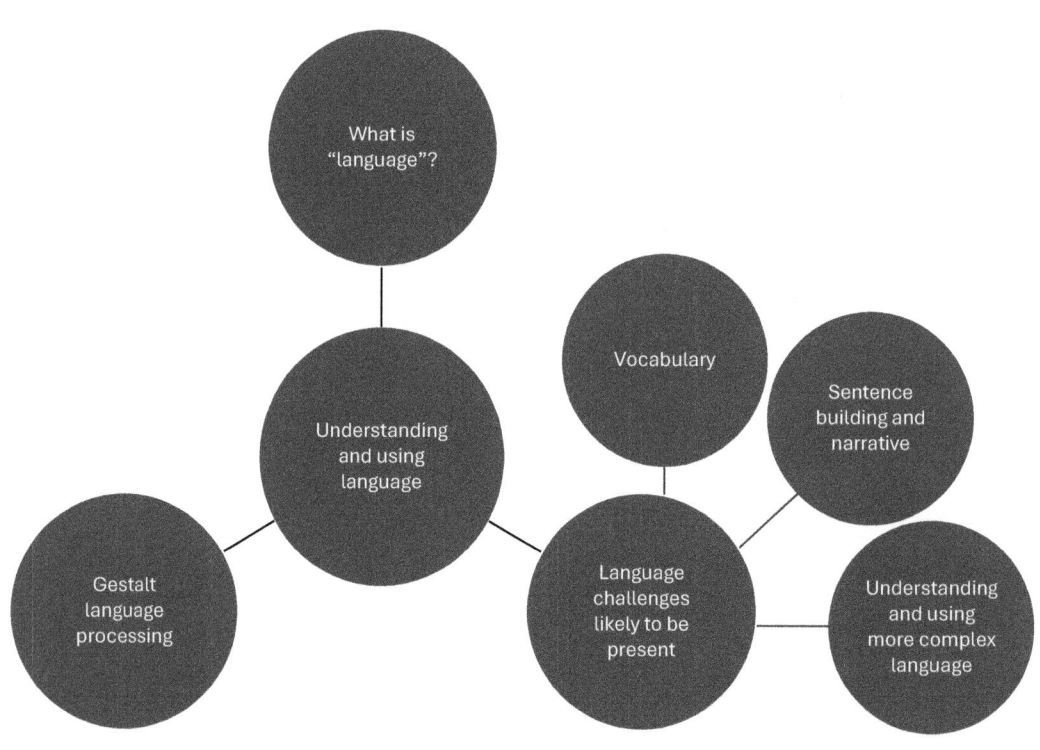

DOI: 10.4324/9781041054986-10

🎯 CHAPTER OBJECTIVES

This chapter focuses on the language we use within teaching, how we embed language teaching within the curriculum and how we can, as educators, identify children that are finding understanding and use of language challenging. It:

- reflects on language learning in terms of use and understanding, further explored in the areas of vocabulary, narrative and language complexity;
- enables you to reflect on your experience of working with children with challenges developing language skills;
- explores the literature and theory related to language learning;
- identifies strategies and key resources to help support pupil's language understanding and use.

Introduction

Developing spoken language is essential for the academic progress of all children. Levels of vocabulary, comprehension and use of sentences have been shown to be a significant indicator of GCSE success in English language, English literature and mathematics (Spencer et al., 2017). This chapter will enable readers to understand the reasons for this association and how to improve outcomes for students by embedding strategies within the curriculum.

🚩 STARTING POINTS

- When giving the children and young people (CYP) you work with verbal instructions, how can you be sure they are able to understand and respond?
- How do you select the words you use?
- How can you check that children and young people understand them sufficiently?
- Do they have the abstract language ability to understand the type of question or instruction given?
- Are they able to respond using the correct words and are they able to combine these to form coherent sentences and narratives?

What is language?

Language includes our knowledge of words and what they mean (semantics), the rules of constructing phrases and sentences (syntax) as well as planning and assembling narratives.

It involves both language understanding (receptive language) and language use (expressive language).

Although this chapter mostly focuses on verbal communication, we also need to acknowledge that a child's language abilities impact both verbal and written communication (see Chapter 8). If a child has a limited vocabulary and finds it challenging to understand long, complex sentences then this will inevitably influence their ability in literacy.

Many factors can impact upon a child's capacity to learn language. We need to consider a CYP's hearing levels and if we have concerns, ensure that a referral is made to have a hearing check. Often CYP, even without hearing difficulties, may find the auditory environment of the classroom difficult and this is something to consider when a child is struggling to keep up with verbal instructions and conversations in the classroom.

 CASE STUDY

David, KS2 primary school teacher and senior lecturer in primary education

Anya was a 7-year-old girl with a diagnosis of Glue Ear. Anya was at times reserved, lacked confidence and reluctant to build friendships with others. It was apparent that Anya was presenting difficulty learning to read at a level expected for her age, there were examples of difficulties with speech and language (mispronunciation of words, missing words in sentences and limited vocabulary) and regular absence from school due to ear infections. Anya was also a little anxious in social situations and quiet in group environments. At times Anya appeared distant, lacking focus and an ability to follow task instructions.

Generating a strong relationship with Anya's mother was invaluable. This dialogue provided me with regular updates regarding emotions, feedback from medical appointments and practical strategies that Anya was comfortable using. I also conducted my own independent research, often consulting information offered by Deafness Research UK and the National Deaf Children's Society.

After being made aware of Anya's situation I was conscious of my approach, teaching style and pedagogy in order to make learning accessible. Some strategies I implemented included:

- Placing Anya where she maintained an unobstructed view of my face. This included talking directly to her at eye level when working 1:1 and encouraging her to listen with her eyes (watch my lip movements when talking). I read Anya's facial expressions and body language carefully when listening to her responses. This helped me understand her spoken word if certain words were not pronounced correctly.

- I would often say 'Anya' prior to starting a conversation. This enabled her to become alert to the fact I was addressing her, enabling Anya to 'fine tune' her listening skills, be prepared for the language used and be ready to focus on instructions.

- I would regularly refer to visual cues such as a 'Now & Next board' and visual timetables to help ensure instructions were precise to help support a clear understanding. In addition to this, sentence frames, manipulatives and emotion graphics were used to help alleviate the reliance on verbal language.
- When communicating collectively as a class, I would often summarise key points, carefully selecting the vocabulary and sentence complexity used to prevent the possibility of cognitive overload.

The strategies I developed through experiences with Anya served me well and enabled me to grow better as a whole educator not just someone supporting a child with a difficulty understanding language. This included being increasingly aware of my positioning in the classroom, giving appropriate visual or oral clues, speaking clearly at a steady pace and avoiding moving around the classroom when talking, all of which help all children, not just those with language difficulties.

The experience with Anya taught me about the importance of building positive and sustained relationships with parents, bridging the home-school gap so that the child knows school and parents are working in tandem for them to achieve the best possible solutions. Although there is a plethora of knowledge and research available, every child is unique and offers a range of preferences and unique requirements. It is important to invest time in knowing the child as an individual, appreciate their struggles and pave a way forward together.

⑦ Critical questions

- How can you improve your communication to assist CYP with language difficulties?
- How can you use the knowledge, understanding and expertise of the parent to improve your own professional development?
- Identify where you can go and who you can talk to support your understanding.
- Consider how language difficulties can have an impact on social situations and behaviour.

When language challenges are likely to be present

CYP can have difficulties acquiring language for many reasons but there are a large number of CYP who have a specific difficulty in developing their understanding and use of language. These CYP may benefit from a diagnosis of Developmental Language Disorder (DLD), which can be diagnosed by a speech and language therapist (SaLT). DLD impacts 7.5% of school age children, which equates to two children in every class (Norbury et al., 2016). CYP with DLD may present with difficulties in multiple areas of language understanding and use, such as understanding words or sentences, word-finding and combining words to make narratives, and pragmatic areas of language such as conversation initiation and maintenance (Bishop et al., 2017). CYP with DLD will present with ongoing challenges and are unlikely to improve without significant support across the key stages, as language complexity and expectations increase. Please see the RADLD (Raising Awareness of DLD) webpages for more information and strategies for the classroom to help support pupils with DLD: https://radld.org/

Vocabulary

Vocabulary has been long regarded as one of the biggest indicators of academic success in core subjects such as English, science and perhaps more surprisingly, maths (Snowling et al., 2011). However, when you consider the abstract concepts that CYP need to have embedded to access even the foundation maths GCSE paper (examples found from one paper include: *decimal, fraction, factorise, obtuse, plot, coordinate, equation, frequency, probability, simultaneous*) then the link becomes more obvious.

It is important to establish that receptive vocabulary (words that CYP understand and have knowledge of) and expressive vocabulary (words that CYP use) should be considered when focusing on strategies and activities designed around vocabulary learning. Often a CYP may understand a word but not use it or conversely use a word in an utterance with very little understanding of what it means.

The first step to consider when we are aiming to teach vocabulary is the selection of target words to focus on. Consider the three tiers of vocabulary framework (Beck et al., 2013, Table 7.1).

So, when selecting words for vocabulary-focused teaching, try to select a combination of Tier 2 and Tier 3 words that will be used throughout the teaching of a particular topic with

Table 7.1 *Summary of the three tiers of vocabulary with examples*

Tier 1 Words	The simplest and most common words, these are mainly learnt through natural conversation and do not usually require specific teaching	*table, cup, rain, climb, big*
Tier 2 Words	These are words that are cross-curricular, more complex but don't tend to be used in general conversation. These are key terms for learning and are often quite abstract. **Tier 3 words are often explained using Tier 2 vocabulary and so pupils who find these difficult will also fail to understand the Tier 3 words.**	*verify, formulate, isolated, diverse, motive, capture, regulate, sparse*
Tier 3 Words	Are often subject specific and are, traditionally, the words focused on when teaching key vocabulary for a topic. Tier 3 words are often prevalent in the language spoken by scientists, musicians and mathematicians.	*parentheses, cardinal, endothermic, baroque*

(Based on Beck et al., 2013).

an emphasis on Tier 2 words. Plan explicit teaching of these target words within topic planning.

There has been a growing consensus of what constitutes effective vocabulary teaching; Graves (2016) summarises this as an environment that is language rich, has direct teaching of word meaning and involves active and meaningful use by CYP of newly taught vocabulary.

There are many resources that can aid with the planning of the delivery of direct teaching of topic vocabulary (see signposting for resources at the end of the chapter). However, there are established strategies and considerations that are key to vocabulary instruction.

- Teach all aspects of a word – not just meaning or a definition. Focus on the sounds in the word, categorise it, encourage pupils to use it in a sentence, write it down. This activity could be at the start of each session for all pupils.
- For pupils needing extra focus on vocabulary learning, words could be **pre-taught** in small groups before the main teaching session. This will mean they have some level of knowledge of the selected focused vocabulary and may be more likely to contribute to whole class activities. (See the resources section for some high-quality resources to help support vocabulary learning across the key stages.)
- Include a **variety of word types**, not just nouns but prepositions, adjectives, verbs and adverbs. These are often the most prevalent within Tier 2 and 3 vocabulary.
- Use **multi-sensory learning** – visuals, actions, drawing, sounds, get your pupils to act out the word.
- **Teach concepts one at a time**, try not to teach opposites at the same time as often these can get confused if you do so. (e.g. on vs not on. Off vs not off. Then on vs off).
- **Teach semantically related words** (e.g. maths vocab for addition, etc.) and the word in its different forms (e.g. prefixes/suffixes).
- **Review taught words regularly**, perhaps have a pot with all focused words in it that gets added to each day. At the end of the week, draw out words at random and ask pupils to formulate a sentence containing that word.

Sentence building and narrative

Understanding language is more than the sum of its parts, and to truly understand and use language effectively, we need to be able to use our life experiences and knowledge of the world. This is known as 'top-down' processing of language (Bishop, 1997, 2014).

It is only with this ability that CYP can accurately understand the language they hear and express their thoughts to others. 'Bottom-up' processes include our knowledge of vocabulary (semantics), word order and grammar (syntax), and knowledge of the social aspects of when and how to talk (pragmatics). At the same time, we use our knowledge and experience of situations, and information from the environment and social context, 'top-down' processes, in order to interpret a speaker's intended meaning. To generate sentences and narratives, we again make use of 'bottom-up' processes – whilst also considering the knowledge and experience of the listener – and use the cues from the listener that identify whether the message has been understood accurately.

CYP with challenges with sentence building and narrative skills may present with difficulties with their receptive (understanding) and expressive skills (use) (Paul et al. 2018; Moraleda-Sepúlveda and López-Resa; 2022), as outlined in Table 7.2 below:

Some strategies that are known to support with sentence and narrative understanding and generation are:

Table 7.2 *How challenges with sentence building and narrative skills might present for CYP and the possible impacts of these on socio-emotional wellbeing*

Receptive	Expressive
• Difficulties identifying key information from conversations, or heard media, e.g. from a story they have listened to, or a TV show or film they have seen • Difficulties summarising or getting the 'gist' • Not following instructions independently – may look to peers and copy, may benefit from information or instructions being repeated	• Speaking in full, 'grammatically correct' sentences – sentences may be short and simple, e.g. contain a single idea or joined by a limited range of connectives, e.g. 'and' • Including determiners such as 'a' and 'the' may not be included, e.g. at the start of sentences or before nouns • Accurately using specific parts of speech, e.g. verbs, prepositions, – so words may not be in the expected order • Changing regular verbs to mark tense (e.g. -ed) or plurality (e.g. -s) (morphological/grammar difficulties) • Structuring ideas, e.g. retelling events or talking about things in chronological order
Possible impacts on socio-emotional wellbeing	
• Experience not being understood, which may lead to frustration or impact on self-esteem and wellbeing. • May be at risk as they may not be able to share their experiences, e.g. if they needed to make a safeguarding disclosure or describe a bullying incident. • If aware of their difficulties, may actively speak in short utterances to maximise their understandability to the listener or may avoid certain speaking situations such as asking for help in the classroom. • Experience social isolation due to not being able to keep up and join in with social banter or share their experiences. • Also have difficulties in their writing (see Chapter 8 for a discussion about the link between language and literacy).	

- Focus on key wh- questions to support the understanding and use of key elements of sentences or narratives, e.g. 'who', 'doing', 'when', 'where' and 'feelings' with visual support, e.g. use of symbols, Makaton signing, coding, e.g. Colourful Semantics (Bryan, 1997) or Shape Coding (Ebbels, 2007). This can be done with the whole class in relation to class texts, or events that have happened/are going to happen.
- Using **multi-sensory learning** (as with vocabulary teaching) may also be beneficial and can be used to support verbal activities as well as written ones (see Figure 7.1).
- **Graphical organisers** to support the development/understanding of sequences and longer narratives (see Figure 7.2 for some examples).
- Regular opportunities for CYP to **share news**, e.g. talk about what happened at the weekend or the evening before, watching age-appropriate news clips, e.g. BBC Newsround and talking about the stories observed, with visual support to talk about 'wh-' questions (as outlined above).
- **Refer to speech and language therapy** – may be able to advise/model specific interventions, e.g. use of coding in order to explicitly teach different elements of sentences or narratives.

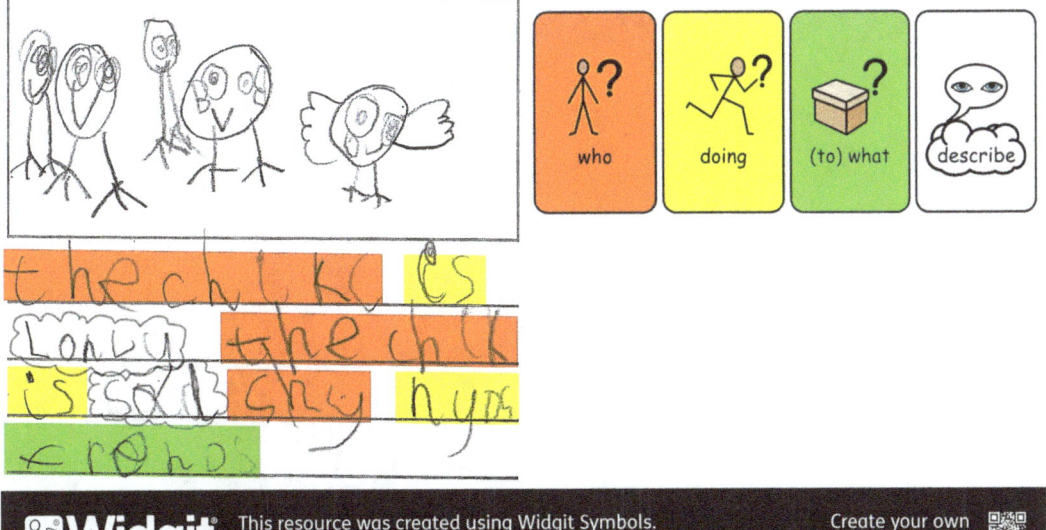

Figure 7.1 *How colour coding and use of symbols can support CYP to identify different elements of sentences, based on Colourful Semantics and Shape Coding. Writing states:* The chick is lonely. The chick is sad. She needs friends. *Although this is a written example, visual coding can also be used to support verbal exchanges. (Permission to reproduce the Widgit Symbols © Widgit Software Ltd. 2002–2025 granted by Anna Cawrey, Partnerships Manager, Widgit, March 2025)*

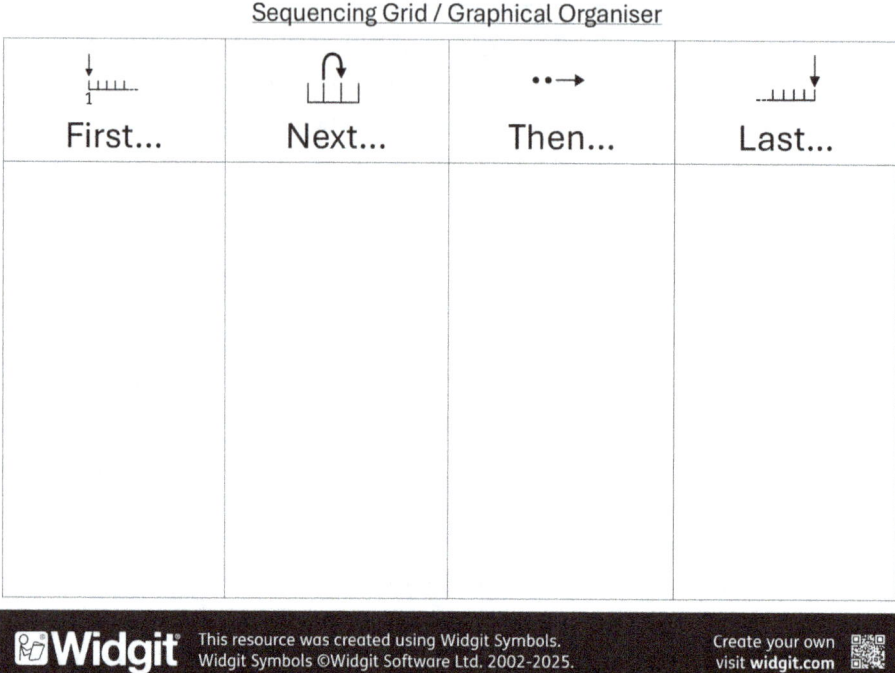

(a)

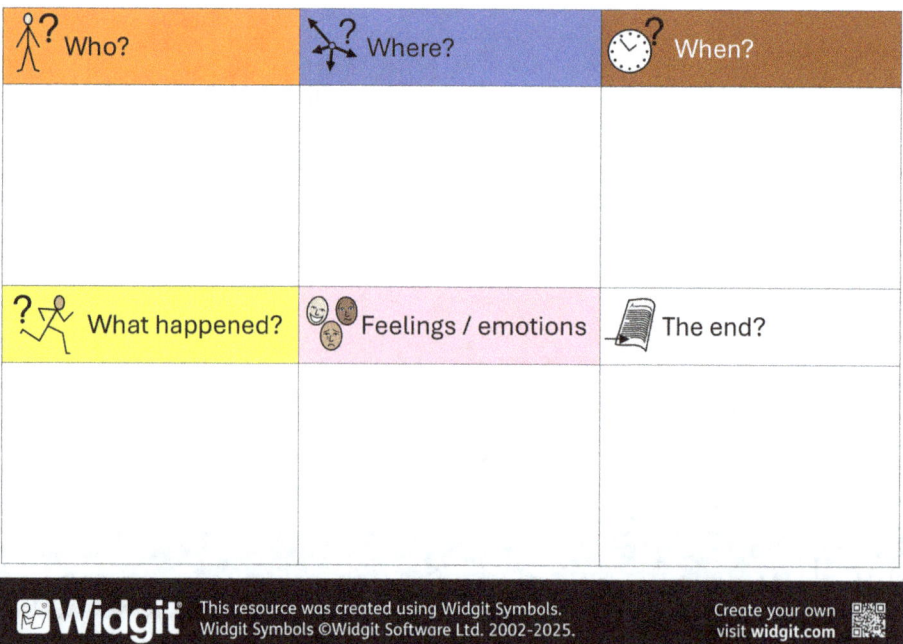

(b)

Figure 7.2 *Example graphical organisers to support sequencing (top) and narrative (bottom) (Permission to reproduce the Widgit Symbols © Widgit Software Ltd. 2002–2025 granted by Anna Cawrey, Partnerships Manager, Widgit, March 2025)*

Understanding and using more complex language

Being able to use 'top-down' processing becomes increasingly key as children move through primary to secondary school, in order to meet the academic demands of the curriculum and also to understand and contribute to social interactions and banter (see Chapter 12). By developing their linguistic skills, children and young people are able to make sense of language that is not explicitly stated and use the cognitively demanding and so-called 'higher-level' language skills of:

- prediction;
- inference;
- problem-solving;
- reasoning;
- understanding the perspective of another;
- understanding and using non-literal and multi-meaning language (such as is required for understanding puns and jokes that rely on word play).

Many educators are familiar with Bloom's taxonomy (Bloom, 1956, updated by Anderson et al., 2001), which characterises aspects of teaching into six areas, increasing in cognitive demand. In speech and language therapy, a different categorisation is used: Blank's levels of questions (Blank, Rose and Berlin, 1978). This is a system that can be used alongside Bloom's but considers the complexity of language at four levels in relation to the context (see Figure 7.3).

The simplest questions (Blank's Level 1) are those that are 'concrete' in nature, that is, they are based on what can be seen or experienced in the here and now. The most challenging questions (Blank's Level 4) are 'abstract', meaning that an individual is required to make use of their knowledge of the world and things in it in order to answer them successfully.

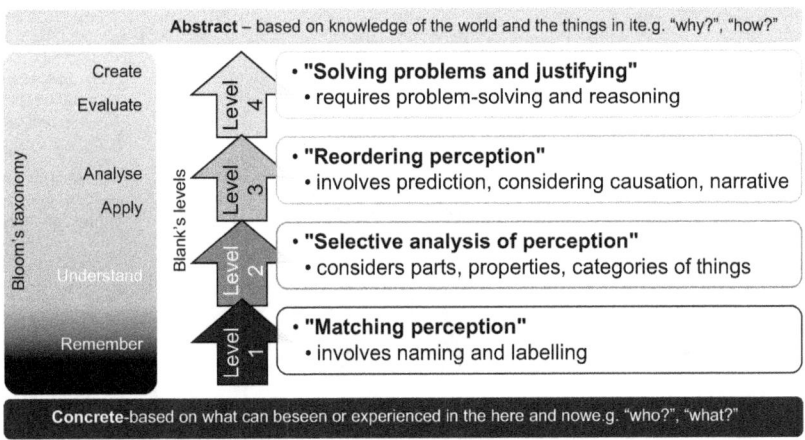

Figure 7.3 Bloom's taxonomy (Anderson et al., 2001) mapped to Blank's levels. (based on Blank, Rose & Berlin, 1978 and Elks & McLachlan, 2008)

Having understanding at Blank's Level 4 is typically assumed in the British education system from Key Stage 1 upwards and indeed having understanding at this level is vital for successful social interaction, emotional understanding and empathising, telling stories/recounting events, understanding the motivations of others, to name a few, however, it is clear that many children and young people are not able to access language at this level. Adults can often be fooled by those CYP who have learnt the format for responding to questions, e.g. they may know that a 'why?' question is answered with 'because...', however, deeper analysis of their response can give an indication of whether they are truly able to understand, manipulate and formulate language at Blank's Level 4.

McLachlan (2025) has recently expanded the Blank's scheme with the addition of Level 5, which children in UK Key Stage 2 and above may demonstrate. At Level 5, CYP are able to apply the skills at Level 4 to novel situations (real and imaginary) that are not being experienced in the here and now, communicate their ideas to others, and work effectively within a group.

The very 'higher-level' nature of language processing also means that our emotions and alertness levels can significantly impact on the capacity to understand and use language at Blank's Levels 3, 4 and 5 (see Chapter 4). Due to the cognitive effort required, when people are stressed/anxious/emotionally dysregulated in some way, the ability to process language and apply the higher-level language skills reduces significantly. Staff supporting children and young people should be aware of this and adapt their language and questions accordingly, depending on the emotional state of the listener. Figure 7.4 demonstrates how adults can adapt their language and use of questions for children and young people of any age.

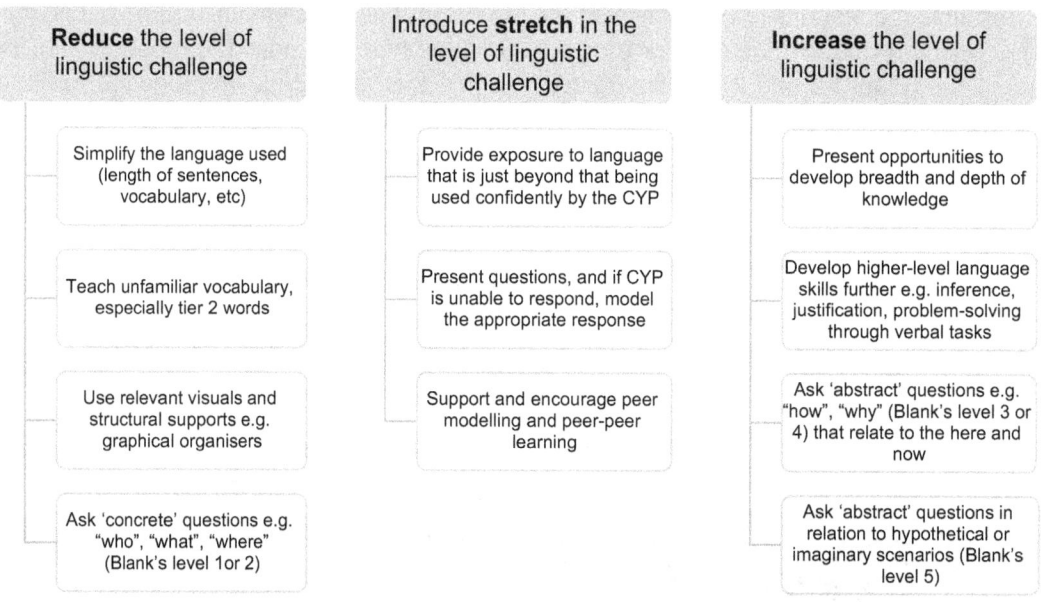

Figure 7.4 Strategies/adaptations for supporting understanding and use of language, including 'higher-level' language

SPOTLIGHT ON EMERGING DEBATES: GESTALT LANGUAGE PROCESSING

Gestalt language processing (GLP) was first discussed in the 1970s but is currently gaining traction both in published literature and in clinical practice. There is currently debate about GLP – its existence and the processes that might be involved, for example, see Hutchins et al. (2024), but education staff, SaLTs and parents are increasingly discussing GLP and the associated implications for supporting CYP.

The ideas and approaches we have described thus far are based on the traditional understanding of language processing, whereby language is built up from word units, to phrases, to sentences, to longer utterances. This is sometimes referred to as 'analytic' language processing. GLP proposes a different way of processing language (e.g. Peters, 1983; Prizant, 1983; Blanc, 2012) whereby language is initially processed in 'chunks' (*gestalts*, or units of meaning) related to a context. The gestalts are then used meaningfully/repeated in other situations (delayed echolalia) that have some link or relation to the context where the gestalt was originally heard. The gestalt is typically uttered with the same intonation and accent as the source. GLP is most commonly noticed in autistic individuals and it is currently believed that episodic memory may have a key role in laying down the gestalts in response to personally meaningful moments (e.g. Prizant, 2012). Over time, the gestalts can be changed or 'mitigated' by the individual and this is the start of the development of self-constructed utterances and grammar with the eventual generation of novel combinations of language. It is important to note that GLP is not a diagnosis, but rather an acknowledgement that language may be being processed and used meaningfully in a non-traditional/non-'analytic' manner.

In practice, education staff and parents may notice that children or young people are frequently repeating back phrases that can be identified from their favoured TV programmes, games or books, although it can be challenging to identify the source of gestalts as they could be from any meaningful interaction, e.g. something that someone has said to them. An even greater challenge is identifying the intended meaning behind the gestalt. For example, a child who is passionate about the Disney Pixar movie *Toy Story* might use the gestalt "To infinity and beyond", which could mean any number of things such as, *I am ready to go now*, or *I'm really enjoying this activity*, or *I want to run*, or *I want my Buzz Lightyear toy*.

If you suspect that a CYP you are working with might be processing language using gestalts, focus on building your relationship with them and on their intended meaning rather than language content. Work collaboratively with parents and colleagues to identify the source of gestalts and therefore the intended meaning. Acknowledge and affirm the use of the gestalts as meaningful communication. When interacting with the individual, follow the CYP's lead and interests. A recent systematic review (Bryant et al., 2024) has found that interventions specifically designed for GLP are not effective and the authors note caution in the use of these, however, current best practice in the UK suggests that working in an individual-led way is likely to promote the best outcomes (e.g. Driver & McLachlan, 2024). Always refer to speech and language therapy if additional guidance is required.

CHAPTER SUMMARY

Language processing is complex but as educators we can play a key role in supporting the development of receptive and expressive skills. This may be in relation to the 'bottom-up' skills of vocabulary and sentence understanding and generation, or 'top-down' skills of understanding context and using 'higher-level' language processes. In doing so, we can enable CYP to participate fully in learning and the social world.

Further reading/resources

- Developmental Language Disorder (DLD) educational support – Speech and Language UK: Changing young lives. See https://speechandlanguage.org.uk/educators-and-professionals/dld-educational-support/ (Accessed 27 August 2025) – contains a downloadable support guide for teachers.
- The Word Aware series of books (Parsons and Branagan, 2021) has developed to support whole class and small group teaching of vocabulary across EYFS, KS1 and 2. See: http://thinkingtalking.co.uk/word-aware/ – Parsons and Branagan (2005) also produced a resource book based on Blank's levels to help CYP across key stages – https://thinkingtalking.co.uk/language-for-thinking/ (accessed 21 March 2025).
- For secondary pupils, please see the amazing resource book by Joffe and Lowe (2022): https://www.taylorfrancis.com/books/mono/10.4324/9780429433177/enriching-vocabulary-secondary-schools-victoria-joffe-hilary-lowe (accessed 21 March 2025).
- For accessible online resources that cover vocabulary packs across national curriculum subjects and free Tier 2 word of the day resources, see: https://vocabularyninja.co.uk/product-category/vocabulary/.
- For more information about using Colourful Semantics please have a look at this fantastic book which aims to support its use and includes access to some practical online resources https://www.routledge.com/Colourful-Semantics-A-Resource-for-Developing-Childrens-Spoken-and-Written-Language-Skills/ForthValley/p/book/9780367210502 (accessed 21 March 2025).

- *Inclusive teamwork for pupils with speech, language and communication needs* outlines a framework for teaching authentic team-working and higher-level language skills for CYP aged seven and above: Merrick, R. (2022). *Inclusive teamwork for pupils with speech, language and communication needs*. Routledge. https://doi.org/10.4324/9781003201717 (accessed 8 April 2025).
- Please see the following YouTube video from Marge Blanc on how to make sense of delayed echolalia Gestalt language processors: https://www.youtube.com/live/eVgTud-IhQA?si=YAZQ8ICX-Pgp_OOA (accessed 21 March 2025).
- For a whole host of resources including guidance and workbooks on GLP, Colourful Semantics and Blanks Levels, please visit: https://s3.elklan.co.uk/Shop/ (accessed 21 March 2025). Elklan also provide accredited training on supporting language and communication skills for CYP of all ages in a range of educational settings.

References

Anderson, L W, Krathwohl, D R and Bloom, B S (2001) *A Taxonomy for Learning, Teaching, and Assessing: A Revision of Bloom's Taxonomy of Educational Objectives*. Boston, MA: Allyn & Bacon.

Beck, I L, McKeown, M G and Kucan, L (2013) *Bringing words to life: Robust vocabulary instruction*. London. Guilford Press.

Bishop, D V M (1997) Cognitive neuropsychology and developmental disorders: Uncomfortable bedfellows. *The Quarterly Journal of Experimental Psychology: Section A*, 50(4): 899–923.

Bishop, D V M (2014) *Uncommon Understanding: Development and Disorders of Language Comprehension in Children*. Hove: Psychology Press.

Bishop, D V M, Snowling, M J, Thompson, P A, Greenhalgh, T and the CATALISE-2 Consortium (2017), Phase 2 of CATALISE: A multinational and multidisciplinary Delphi consensus study of problems with language development: Terminology. *Journal of Child Psycholgy and Psychiatry*, 58(10): 1068–1080.

Blanc, M (2012) *Natural Language Acquisition on the Autism Spectrum: The Journey from Echolalia to Self-Generated Language*. Madison, WI: Communication Development Center.

Blank, M, Rose, S A and Berlin, L J (1978). *The Language of Learning: The Preschool Years*. New York: Grune and Stratton.

Bloom, B S (1956) *Taxonomy of Educational Objectives, Handbook: The Cognitive Domain*. New York: David McKay.

Bryan, A (1997) Colourful semantics. In Chiat, S, Law, J and Marshall, T (eds.). *Language Disorders in Children and Adults: Pscholoinguistic Approaches to Therapy*. London: Whurr.

Bryant, L, Bowen, C, Grove, R, Dixon, G, Beals, K, Shane, H and Hemsley, B (2024) Systematic review of interventions based on gestalt language processing and natural language acquisition (glp/nla): clinical implications of absence of evidence and cautions for clinicians and parents. *Current Developmental Disorders Reports*, 12(1): 1–14.

Driver, H and McLachlan, H (2024) *Language Builders for Gestalt Language Processors*. St. Mabyn: Elklan.

Ebbels, S (2007) Teaching grammar to school-aged children with specific language impairment using shape coding. *Child Language Teaching and Therapy*, 23(1): 67–93.

Elks, L and McLachlan, H (2008) *Language Builders*. St. Mabyn: Elklan.

Graves, M F, (2016) *The Vocabulary Book: Learning and Instruction* (2nd ed). London: Teachers College Press.

Hutchins T L, Knox S E and Fletcher E C (2024) Natural language acquisition and gestalt language processing: A critical analysis of their application to autism and speech language therapy. *Autism and Developmental Language Impairments*. 22(9):1–20.

Joffe, V and Lowe, H (2022) *Enriching Vocabulary in Secondary Schools: A Practical Resource for Teachers and Speech and Language Therapists*. London. Routledge.

McLachlan, H (2025) *The Blank Language Scheme Revisited*. St. Mabyn: Elklan.

Moraleda-Sepúlveda, E and López-Resa, P (2022) Morphological difficulties in people with developmental language disorder. *Children* 9(2):125.

Norbury C F, Gooch D, Wray C, Baird G, Charman T, Simonoff E, Vamvakas G and Pickles A (2016) The impact of nonverbal ability on prevalence and clinical presentation of language disorder: evidence from a population study. *Journal of Child Psychology and Psychiatry*. 57(11):1247–1257.

Parsons, S and Branagan, A (2005) *Language for thinking: A Structured Approach for Young Children*. Milton Keynes: Speechmark.

Parsons, S and Branagan, A (2021) *Word Aware 1: Teaching Vocabulary Across the Day, Across the Curriculum* (2nd edition.). London: Routledge.

Paul, R, Norbury, C and Gosse, C (2018) *Language Disorders from Infancy Through Adolescence: Speaking Listening, Reading, Writing, Communicating* 5th edition. St Louis: Mosby Elsevier.

Peters, A M (1983) *The Units of Language Acquisition, Cambridge Monographs and Texts in Applied Psycholinguistics*. Cambridge: Cambridge University Press.

Prizant, B (1983) Language acquisition and communicative behaviour in Autism: Toward an understanding of the "whole" of it. *Journal of Speech and Hearing Disorders*, 48(3): 296–307.

Prizant, B M (2012) The power of emotional memory. *Autism Spectrum Quarterly* 17:37–38. https://barryprizant.com/wp-content/uploads/2015/07/asq17_power_of_emotional_memory_spring_2012.pdf

Snowling, M J, Hulme, C, Bailey, A M, Stothard, S. and Lindsay, G (2011) Language and literacy attainment of pupils during early years and through key stage 2: does teacher assessment at five provide a valid measure of children's current and future educational attainments? *Better Communication Research Programme*, Department for Education. Available at: https://dera.ioe.ac.uk/id/eprint/13689/ (accessed 21 March 2025).

Spencer, S, Clegg, J, Stackhouse, J and Rush, R (2017) Contribution of spoken language and socio-economic background to adolescents' educational achievement at age 16 years. *International Journal of Language and Communication Disorders*, 52(2): 184–196.

8 Literacy and language

Tom Hopkins and Natacha Capener

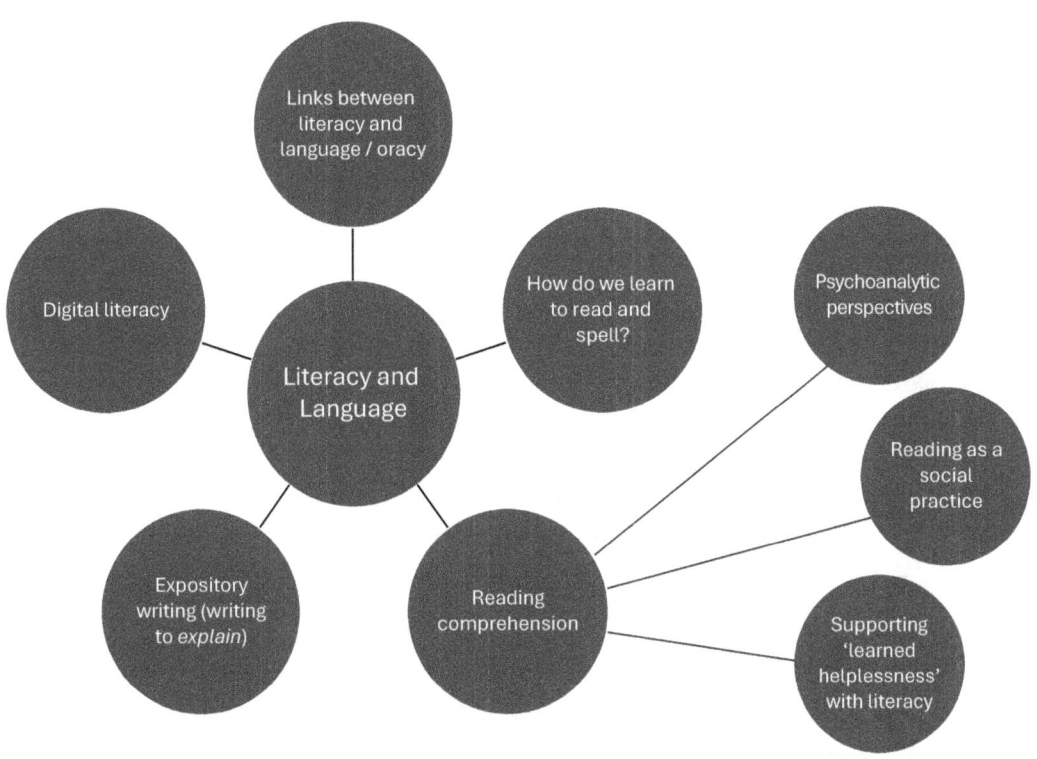

⊙ CHAPTER OBJECTIVES

This chapter explores the links between language and literacy. The chapter:

- Explains why speech and language therapists may have a role in some elements of literacy.

- Discusses the links between literacy and language with reference to theory, considering both psycholinguistic and socio-cultural aspects of reading comprehension, as well as writing for different purposes.

- Considers the observable clues that might indicate whether a child or young person has difficulties with language that are impacting on their reading and writing.

- Outlines some ideas for supporting language in the educational environment that will impact on the child/young person's reading and writing skills, including how speech and language therapists and education staff can work collaboratively in this.

As Snow (2016: 219) states

> The transition to literacy is a linguistic achievement, building on the psycholinguistic competencies (phonemic awareness, expressive and receptive vocabulary, narrative language skills and so on) that children bring to school and augmenting these with best-practice classroom instructional approaches that foster the child's ability to transition from a biologically "natural" code (talking and listening) to one that is biologically "unnatural", but of enormous social, political, cultural and economic importance.

⚑ STARTING POINTS

- What do you already know about the link between reading and/or writing and spoken language?

- What aspects of learning to read and write might have something to do with oracy?

- How do you support your pupils to develop their literacy skills? Do any of these strategies also develop their understanding and/or use of language?

Introduction: Links between literacy and language/oracy

Let's start by discussing what we mean by the term 'literacy'. Here we are considering:

- word reading and the skills it encompasses (i.e. phonological awareness (PA) and decoding – see Chapter 6 where PA is discussed in more detail);
- spelling (aka re-coding);

- reading comprehension (the understanding of text and related skills including inferencing and world knowledge);
- writing (motor skills and the cognitive process of idea generation and planning).

So, why would speech and language therapists (SaLTs) have anything to do with literacy? The same structures underpinning the skills required for language and communication are involved in reading and writing, at least for the majority of people. These linguistic/oracy elements are often the cause of difficulties which may first be noticed by education staff as difficulties with reading and writing (literacy).

As outlined in more detail in Chapter 7, research shows two pupils out of 30 in a class are likely to have pervasive, long-term difficulties with language understanding and use which will require specialist intervention from a SaLT (Norbury et al., 2016). These pupils are highly likely to also have reading and writing challenges that may persist into adulthood (Whitehouse et al. 2009).

In this chapter, we are not focusing on the physical motor skills required for writing and letter formation (we would advise getting support from occupational therapists for this). We will instead focus on the top-down, psycholinguistic processes (see Chapter 7) that support children in reading, both in fluency and comprehension, as well as being able to convert sounds to print to generate/structure ideas for writing. We are also not focusing on dyslexia per se, but describe the presentation of common reading and writing difficulties and how these can be supported.

Unlike spoken language, literacy is considered to be biologically secondary knowledge. This means exposure alone does not result in sufficient knowledge output and explicit instruction is therefore required (Snow, 2016). Educators must therefore be confident in the processes and skills making up literacy and how to support them. It is also why phonics programmes provide explicit systematic instruction to support children's decoding skills. This psycholinguistic approach to literacy is rather different to an approach which views literacy as a social practice embedded in socio-cultural rituals. The latter perspective is important for us to consider when implementing literacy practice with children as they are more likely to engage in literacy activities shared with other members of their community that relate to their own interests, values and identities. In fact, literacy can and should be used as a means to provide exploration of these.

> ### ⓘ CRITICAL QUESTIONS
>
> - What do I already understand about the link between literacy and language?
> - Am I already supporting the development of literacy skills via oracy?
> - What do I want the learner(s) to access from the texts they are provided with? What do I need to change about lesson delivery to make this happen?
> - What am I doing to engage learners in reading and writing activities? How can I link activities to their socio-cultural backgrounds and real-life experience?

How do we learn to read and spell?

Phonological awareness (PA), as outlined in Chapter 6, has been consistently recognised as a strong predictor of reading ability in young children and such evidence has influenced policy and practice via the inclusion of phonics reading programmes in schools (Castles et al., 2018). Phonics are often systematic in their approach to supporting children to 'break the code' as they begin learning the correct grapheme to phoneme correspondences (GPC) (matching the letters to the sounds) and then how to write these (orthographical knowledge). Phonics will focus initially on the teaching of regular, transparent GPCs that children are exposed to more frequently. However, the English language is considered a deep orthographic language, which means it contains words considered 'irregular' because they do not conform to the typical GPC rules children are exposed to. In fact, approximately 50% of words in English do not conform to the GPC rules (Devonshire, et al. 2013). Children are likely to mispronounce irregular words like 'bear', the', or 'pint' when they decode using the more common/typical GPC rules they encounter. Furthermore, many words have the same pronunciation but are spelled differently (two, too) and some words like 'lead' have different pronunciations depending on the context (homophones). Given there is more regularity in the morphological makeup of English words, providing morphological training/instruction to children early on in their literacy journey can support them in reading and spelling these irregular words. Despite stage theories of reading development suggesting morphological instruction should come later, studies have shown children as young as five years can use morphology to aid their reading and spelling (Devonshire et al., 2013). This advocates for teachers to include information about the written form of English and how it works. The more exposure children have reading via GPC and morphological instruction, the less they rely on the laboured process of decoding and can instead, draw on their memory of the correct pronunciation of words, particularly those considered irregular (Coltheart, 2005). Novel words or non-words, however, will still require decoding. This is important for educators to realise in any instances where they observe children struggling in their attempt to read new or non-words as well as children who rely too much on their decoding, particularly for familiar, irregular words (see 'What to look out for' section on page 119).

Children also find the spelling of less transparent (irregular) words difficult as they have to re-code the phonological representation of a word or grapheme to its written output. Spelling also requires sufficient motor production to physically write words, and working memory to identify the correct phonemes, followed by the correct graphemes (letters) to match (Moxam, 2020). To aid children in the spelling of irregular words, Moxam (2020) proposes the teaching of semantics and morphology in addition to the application of the GPC rules children encounter via phonics. This is important to consider, as children often make mistakes in their attempt in representing the sounds they hear. Children can instead draw upon their knowledge of consistent morphemes for spelling words in the past tense (-ed) and the meaning of words for the spelling of homophones (two/too/to). Having access to a SaLT means children's spelling errors can be appropriately assessed and analysed to inform target intervention at the semantic, phonological, orthographical and/or morphological level.

Reading comprehension

Psycholinguistic perspectives

The more exposure children have to reading and as their ability to decode increases, the more fluent a reader they are likely to become. At this point, children are afforded the cognitive space to process and infer the meaning behind text, enabling the transition from learning to read to reading to learn (Laberge and Samuels, 1974). Processing and inferring the meaning behind text utilises spoken language skills that include vocabulary, grammatical and morphological knowledge as well as an understanding of the structure of stories (Klauda & Guthrie, 2008). The simple view of reading (Gough & Tunmer, 1986, see Figure 8.1) illustrates the importance of spoken language (aka language comprehension/understanding) and text decoding in understanding what is read.

Figure 8.1 emphasises the unique and equal contribution that both decoding (D) and spoken language comprehension (LC) components have in supporting reading comprehension through a multiplication rather than additive formulae used to signify reading comprehension (RC): D X LC = RC. Neither component, therefore, compensates for weaknesses in the other. So, the reading comprehension abilities of children who have language comprehension difficulties, but superior decoding abilities (fluent reader also known hyperlexic – see 'What to look out for' on page 119), will suffer, because of the limitations in the former. Similarly, children with sufficient language comprehension will demonstrate problems in their reading comprehension should they display accompanying difficulties in their text decoding abilities. Adults who are able to monitor and identify children's language abilities can therefore provide essential insight into children's reading comprehension abilities.

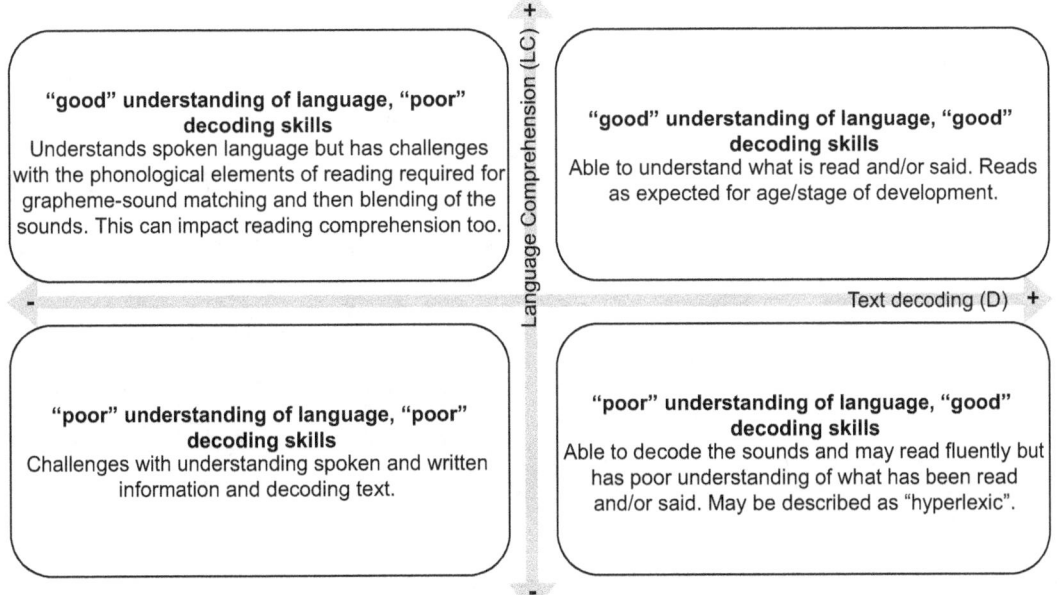

Figure 8.1 *The 'simple' view of reading. Based on Gough & Tunmer (1986)*

Reading as a social practice

During the 1980s, a paradigm shift occurred situating literacy away from the psycholinguistic perspective to one that emphasised literacy as a socio-cultural practice embedded in a wider political context (Unrau et al., 2019). In accordance with this school of thought, literacy is a representation of discourse that reflects specific socio-cultural norms and practices. Research has since delved into exploring differences in literacy practice within contexts, such as the home and school environment with exploration of literacy transformation in line with socio-cultural changes including digital literacies.

Whilst the socio-cultural context is often missing in the psycholinguistic models outlined above, other models, such as Snow's (2002) heuristic for thinking about reading comprehension (see Figure 8.2) include this. Snow's model positions reading within the socio-cultural context, whereby the individual reader's abilities, knowledge and beliefs surrounding reading interact with and are influenced by their environment and the reading activity. In such models, the meaning taken from reading is socially constructed, therefore placing weight on the influence of learning experiences situated at home and within the classroom (Ruddell et al., 2019).

Following on from this perspective, it might be useful to consider strategies to support children in their reading (particularly with comprehension) that incorporate shared reading practices either at home or in the classroom. Dialogic reading is an example of shared reading that promotes a scaffolding approach to reading and has been shown to facilitate both literacy and oral language development (Pillinger & Vardy, 2022). It promotes active involvement and participation of the child in the reading process placing

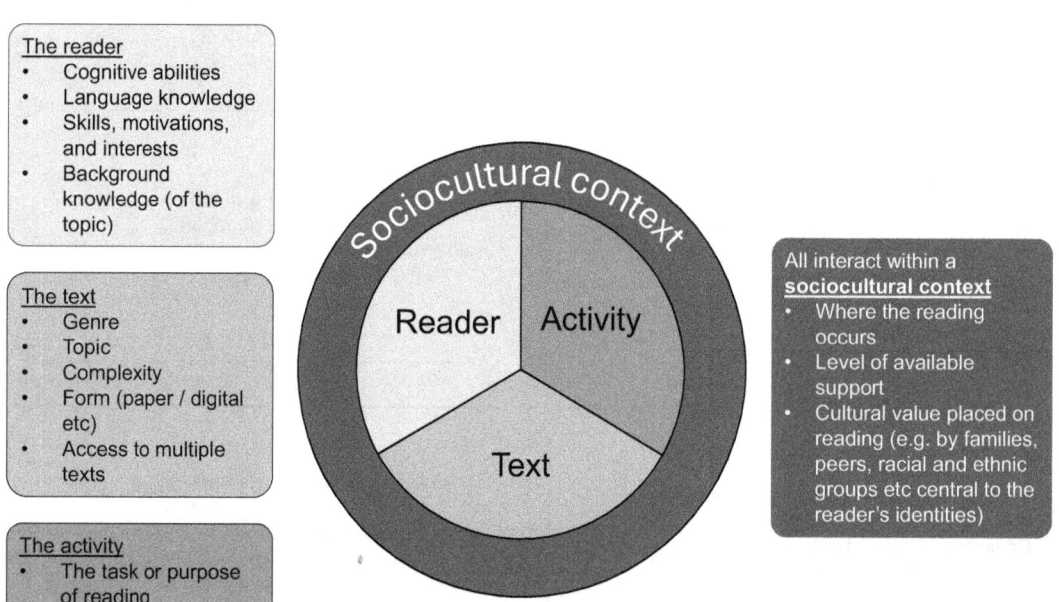

Figure 8.2 Demonstrating the different factors influencing reading comprehension

"adapted from Snow's (2002) heuristic for thinking about reading comprehension, https://www.rand.org/pubs/monograph_reports/MR1465.html, shared with kind permission"

them as the storyteller and the adult the listener. There are parallels that can be drawn between dialogic reading and dialogic teaching that was discussed in Chapter 1.

 Dialogic reading can be promoted using the following strategies during shared reading:

- **The use of prompting** to ask children open 'wh' questions about the book. This can be anything about the characters, a key event or occurrence. You could use any images of the book to help the child consider what might be going on or use prompts to ask children to complete a sentence related to the story (see Chapter 7 for a graphical organiser example which contains key wh- questions/prompts to use).
- **Evaluate the answer** and then **expand on the child's response** by rephrasing or adding more to the answer introducing novel vocabulary as you do.
- Asking the child to **repeat back** by asking again the original prompt.
- It is also good practice to relate aspects of the book to the **child's own lived experience** using the same process above.
- **Repetition** of the same books can help children cement key vocabulary to help develop their language and literacy.

Supporting 'learned helplessness' with literacy in the educational environment

Some children and young people find it difficult to engage in the explicit teaching of literacy, including structured phonics programmes, which can impact their confidence and motivation to want to read. This could result in a belief of not being a good reader and a behaviour of not wanting to pursue related literacy activities.

 Here are some suggestions for how to support children and young people who present with low confidence with reading and writing:

- **Promote a universal ethos that 'every child is a reader'** regardless of background and experience. Some children will come from an environment where literacy plays a big part, whereas others less so and these children, as they enter formal education, may have preconceived notions of literacy and their ability that need to be challenged. Ask children to write or talk about the relevance literacy has to their lives to help instil this belief and culture.

- **Focus literacy activities around the child's socio-cultural identities.** Children may not identify themselves as a 'reader' and may not identify with the books/resources that they are asked to engage in. Consider providing access to a wide range of texts to match the interests and values of the children you support. You could ask children to write about aspects of their own lives and to share these with their peers (along with books they like to read), so other children begin to appreciate the diverse socio-cultural practices of their class, including them in their own literacy activities.

- **Provide choice on what children read and write** to increase motivation and enjoyment in reading. For older children, you might also consider providing a choice for how they write. Note that it is still important to help the child choose texts that align with their skill set (see Chapter 3).

- **Promote intrinsic motivation to read and write.** Be less focused on attainment and external rewards for progress and engagement but focus instead on the activity itself and the benefits this can bring to children now and in the future. This will help children to see the value in reading.

- **Provide regular feedback on process and effort rather than outcome.** Highlight what students are doing well in with regard to their approach to literacy and provide supportive strategies to help them achieve their aims. This will increase self-confidence and self-efficacy.

⑦ CRITICAL QUESTIONS

- How could you use culturally varied and individualised materials to support the reading comprehension of the children and young people you work with?

- How could these also be used or adapted to support engagement in and access to creative writing opportunities?

Expository writing (writing to *explain*)

Writing requires planning ideas around a common theme that are organised to achieve a specific goal. These ideas are then translated into language and then transcribed to text. Once this is done, further editing occurs through a review of the text produced (Flower and Hayes, 1981). Not only do these processes rely on motor and linguistic skills but they also require sufficient cognitive skills (working memory/executive functioning (Nippold and Scott, 2010) – see Chapters 2 and 7), which are especially important for 'high-level' literacy activities that older children (in UK Key Stage 3) are expected to engage in and which place greater demand on executive functioning. Expository writing is an example of this and is present in a range of subjects. It involves writing for purpose and for a target audience that constructs an argument to inform and persuade. Factual evidence is reviewed and evaluated in expository writing through the application of language considered more complex in comparison to conversation (Nippold and Scott, 2010). The complex language involved in expository writing can include:

- The use and understanding of abstract, less frequently used subject-specific vocabulary (semantics)
- Complex grammar used to construct concise clear arguments of which also requires strong narrative skills (syntax).
- The application of poetic licence and strategies, such as metaphor when constructing an attractive, engaging written argument for a particular target audience (metalinguistics).
- Here is an example of expository writing: *Photosynthesis is like a recipe for life, where the main ingredient of sunlight is combined with water and carbon dioxide to create the essential energy plants require to grow*. If you were to talk about photosynthesis in conversation, the tone would likely be more informal and the language simplified.

Knowing that the construction of written discourse requires sufficient language skills means children who struggle with their writing are likely to have related language difficulties that can be identified and supported with the help of professionals such as speech and language therapists.

For younger children who are developing their writing skills, limitations in their writing are to be expected and will reflect common errors found in spoken language. For example, theme muddling (unclear organisation of the ideas) is typically seen in both written and spoken language as young children begin to engage in narrative. Errors in the use of past tense and pronoun use are also common, as are mistakes in the spelling of atypical words that do not confirm to the GPC rules (Perera, 1984). Here is an example of a sentence containing errors considered typical for young children: *Me rund to skool* or *Him sed he goed to the parc*. NB When there is a disparity between spoken and written language or the errors in writing seem to persist, it may be beneficial to seek support.

 SPOTLIGHT ON NEW DEBATE: DIGITAL LITERACY

In today's world, the meaning of being literate is evolving towards multiple literacy which also includes information and communication technologies… the nature of reading and writing is changing. For students to be literate nowadays, they should be able to read hypertexts, use multimedia components and the internet effectively for accessing information and structuring meaning, join various online communities and use various media resources outside the classroom.

(Yamaç, Öztürk, & Mutlu, 2020, p. 2)

Access to computers and technology is now almost universal, so it is important for CYP to have the skills needed for them to be proficient digital citizens. This means that 'knowledge' is readily available to all, and therefore the need for people to hold specific information in memory is reducing, whereas the need to know how to access and use knowledge and information is increasing (McLachlan, 2025). To successfully and safely interact with and learn from digital media, CYP are required to apply higher-level language skills, social cognition, and emotional regulation in addition to their (digital) literacy skills per se. UNESCO (2024) outline five 'domains' important for the development of "ethical digital citizens": digital literacy; safety and resilience; participation and agency; emotional intelligence; and creativity and innovation. Each of the domains require the requisite higher-level language skills we discussed in Chapter 7, and the authors argue that all of these need to be addressed and explicitly taught within school curricula.

Educators can support CYP to develop the following skills in relation to digital content (including that generated by artificial intelligence) by explicitly teaching:

- how to determine fact vs opinion;
- critical thinking (e.g. to determine whether a source is trustworthy, to consider bias, to compare sources);
- independent problem-solving (e.g. in relation to finding required information, generating searches/AI prompts, etc.);
- analysis of risk, including being aware of the risks of communicating with unfamiliar others online or to identify phishing emails (OECD, 2021) as well as keeping themselves safe;
- the social rules or 'netiquette' that apply online/to digital communication and how to apply these;
- how content they share digitally might be perceived by others (perspective taking) and how they manage negative comments received (digital emotional intelligence and social cognition skills);
- creativity and flexibility to adapt to changes in the developing technological landscape.

If these skills are not honed, developed and prioritised throughout childhood and young adulthood, then pupils will not be adequately prepared for their adult lives or the world of work (see Chapter 12).

GUIDANCE FOR ADAPTIVE PLANNING

 What to look out for

There are some signs educators can look out for that may indicate difficulties with reading and writing, which may be caused or exacerbated by an underlying difficulty with language/oracy:

- Displays consistent difficulties in sounding out the sounds of words they hear and/or also letters/words they see in print that you expect them to be decoding. May rely on visual cues of letters and images when attempting to read words.
- Is able to 'read' familiar words by sight (using memory) but not able to apply blending rules to non-words or unfamiliar words.
- Overuses phonetic rules, e.g. uses blending even for words to which they have been exposed many times, particularly for irregular words typically learned by sight/morphology.
- Are able to decode and blend/read fluently but not able to demonstrate comprehension of what is read (may be described as "hyperlexic", Gough & Tunmer, 1986).
- Seem to 'dread' reading aloud.
- Don't like to be chosen to answer questions about what has been read or to give their ideas, e.g. contributions to a story.
- Seem to wait and watch others before starting activities, especially when given written instructions.
- Avoid lessons where reading and writing have a heavy focus, e.g. literacy/English, humanities – this may be asking to go to the toilet a lot in these classes, arriving late or non-attendance.
- Seem verbally able (maybe 'chatty') but are reluctant to engage in literacy tasks or produce written work which does not seem to reflect their verbal skills.
- Always choose a particular reading book/series with which they are very familiar.

This is not an exhaustive list and none of these alone necessarily indicate difficulties with reading and writing, but they may be worth investigating further. Please discuss any concerns with literacy leads and/or the school SENDCo. It may be beneficial to seek out assessment for dyslexia or SLCN.

> **What can I do to help?**
>
> Supporting reading comprehension requires similar strategies to supporting language comprehension (see Chapter 7).
>
> How educators can help children and young people presenting with the difficulties or behaviours described above will depend on several factors, but possibly the most salient of these is the pupil's age or cognitive level (Table 8.1); please also see the strategies that we have included throughout the chapter.

Table 8.1 Strategies to develop language and literacy skills throughout a child/young person's educational journey

Early years (up to end of Reception)	<ul><li>Developing phonological awareness skills to lay the foundations for literacy (see Chapter 6)</li><li>Making adaptations to phonics teaching – considering the child's readiness</li><li>Development of spelling (via decoding and sound-grapheme mapping)</li><li>Exposure to print through shared story time, featuring a range of high-interest and culturally representative topics/materials. Fostering an 'early love of reading'</li><li>Engage in dialogic reading (see strategies above)</li></ul>
Middle years – Key Stage 1 and 2 (Years 1–6)	<ul><li>Building on the recommendations from early years</li><li>Development of vocabulary and 'knowledge' to support reading comprehension (see Chapter 7)</li><li>Development of language structures to support use of context – morphology (word endings to mark tense and plurality, etc.) and syntax (word order and sentence structure) particularly to support comprehension of unfamiliar vocabulary or to determine the 'gist'</li><li>Development of sequencing and narrative skills (see Chapter 7)</li><li>Development of self-monitoring to consider what a reader can understand from what is written</li><li>Supporting confidence, motivation and enjoyment of reading and writing – developing a culture that celebrates reading, values the interests of children and young people, and draws on their own life experience</li><li>Development of digital literacy and associated skills (reading and writing on screen) (see section on 'digital literacy')</li></ul>

Table 8.1 (Continued)

Older pupils – Key Stage 3 and 4 (secondary age and above)	<ul><li>Building on the recommendations for early and middle years</li><li>Developing reading comprehension of abstract/metaphorical meaning in text</li><li>Developing writing stamina</li><li>Development of different forms or styles of writing, e.g. expository writing, writing fiction vs non-fiction</li><li>Development of skill in writing with differing 'voice', including the higher-level language skills of considering the experience of others, e.g. the experience, motivations and emotions of a character (see Chapter 7)</li><li>Explicit teaching prefixes and suffixes in relation to word origins/etymology</li></ul>

Application

Throughout this chapter we have endeavoured to outline how literacy and language are interwoven and have emphasised that supporting the development of language/oracy skills is likely to have a positive impact on reading, reading comprehension, idea generation and writing. In doing so, we hope we have clearly communicated that literacy is best supported when both education professionals and communication professionals (SaLTs) work collaboratively. The following case study demonstrates the rich outcomes that can be achieved when there is scope and freedom for this to happen.

 CASE STUDY

Charlotte, secondary English teacher, inner-city academy setting

Our English department trialled a new approach to teaching: a partnership model of teacher and SaLT co-teaching a small class of Year 10 students who presented with significant SEND across all four categories of need. I took over as the teacher for GCSE and all but one of these eight wonderful young people sat their exams. We had been unsure if GCSEs were the right qualification: we didn't want to set them up for failure but limiting their potential was wrong, so we took a very child-centred approach, relying heavily on speech and language therapy principles and assessing next steps regularly. Students also took AQA's Step Up to English qualification as part of this journey.

Fast forward to August, and the best news arrived: all seven had passed their GCSE, three at the government's 'standard pass' of a four. So, what was the root of their success? Maximising the fact that the school had bought in a full-time SaLT from the NHS.

Teachers' SEND training is often rudimentary. So, we shared planning and delivery and developed each other's knowledge and skills to become more holistic practitioners.

Natacha taught me to use word maps, to use Blank's system of questioning and much more. My expertise was needed to teach the curriculum but I couldn't have taught it as effectively to these students if she wasn't teaching me and working also directly with the students. It required an enormous amount of cooperation and team planning but was well worth it. We devised a highly differentiated curriculum for the group – crucially with a heavy focus on oracy. We didn't always agree but we were committed to listening to each other.

A typical poetry lesson might follow this structure:

- visual schedule of skills such as listening, thinking, writing and speaking;
- SaLT task developing a specific area of language such as inference and prediction, sometimes related to current affairs;
- key vocabulary, using 'word maps';
- class verbal reading and annotation;
- independent thinking time for students to generate and ask questions they had about the story, structure or content of the poem;
- summarising one aspect of learning.

We embarked on this project with a clear goal: to provide the students with the skills required to access and engage with the world around them to the best of their ability. The GCSE passes opened doors to further study but, most importantly, students' confidence and communication developed, bringing them closer to their 'more able' peers.

Having two highly qualified professionals with one class is costly. But we argue it's education, health and care plan funding and staff effort that can't be better spent.

ⓘ Critical questions

- Are there possibilities for collaboration between education and SaLT in your setting?
- If not, how could relationships/collaboration be developed?

📝 CHAPTER CONCLUSION

Language and literacy share underlying processes and so supporting language/oracy also supports literacy, especially in relation to reading comprehension and writing preparation/planning. However, it is not enough to focus on the mechanics of reading, writing or language. A child or young person's socio-cultural context and engagement/motivation are also key to maximising success in both oracy and literacy in the ever-evolving technological world. Educators and SaLTs have unique contributions to bring to the development of literacy skills, and sharing expertise in a practical way can result in broad and positive functional outcomes for children and young people.

📖 Further reading/resources

All weblinks provided below were accessed in March 2025 and correct at time of publishing.

Supporting writing and idea generation

Some existing programmes that have an oracy focus (this is not an exhaustive list and please do your own research before determining which, if any, of these might be suitable for your setting)

- Let's Think in English – https://www.letsthinkinenglish.org/
- Literacy Shed – https://www.literacyshed.com/
- Philosophy 4 Children – https://p4c.com/
- Talk 4 Writing – https://www.talk4writing.com/

A fantastic book about supporting essay writing for adolescents with language and learning difficulties, but the strategies suggested may be applicable to all learners who are having difficulties with essay writing

Knight, K. (2022) *Essay Writing for Adolescents with Language and Learning Difficulties: Practical Strategies for English Teachers* (1st ed.). Routledge. https://doi.org/10.4324/9781003263401

Supporting digital literacy and related skills

UK Government – Department for Education – Information about the 'Connect the Classroom' initiative

https://www.gov.uk/guidance/connect-the-classroom

Literacy Trust – Fake news and critical literacy resources

https://literacytrust.org.uk/resources/fake-news-and-critical-literacy-resources/

UNESCO – Global citizenship education in a digital age: teacher guidelines (2024) – This resource includes lesson plans and strategies for teaching digital skills and critical thinking.

https://unesdoc.unesco.org/ark:/48223/pf0000388812?locale=en

Collaborative working between education and speech and language therapy

Northumbria Healthcare NHS Foundation Trust-Newcastle University Universal, Targeted and Specialist (NNUTS) Framework (Stringer, Nicholson, & Hope, 2024)

https://research.ncl.ac.uk/nnuts/

The Balanced System Framework

https://www.thebalancedsystem.org/

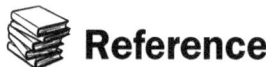# References

Castles, A, Rastle, K, and Nation, K (2018) Ending the reading wars: Reading acquisition from novice to expert. *Psychological Science in the Public Interest*, 19(1): 5–51.

Coltheart, M (2005) Modeling reading: The dual route approach. In Snowling, M J and Hulme, C (2005) *The Science of Reading: A Handbook*. 1st ed. Malden, MA: Blackwell Pub.

Devonshire, V, Morris, P, and Fluck, M (2013) Spelling and reading development: The effect of teaching children multiple levels of representation in their orthography. *Learning and Instruction*, 25: 85–94.

Flower, L and Hayes J R (1981) A cognitive process theory of writing. *College Composition and Communication* 32(4): 365–387.

Gough, P and Tunmer W (1986) Decoding, reading, and reading disability. *Remedial and Special Education*, 7(1): 6–10.

Klauda S L and Guthrie, J T (2008) Relationships of three components of reading fluency to reading comprehension. *Journal of Educational Psychology*, 100(2): 310–321.

Laberge, D and Samuels, S (1974) Toward a theory of automatic information processing in reading. *Cognitive Psychology*, 6(2): 293–323.

McLachlan, H (2025) *The Blank Language Scheme Revisited*. St. Mabyn: Elklan.

Moxam, C (2020) The Link between language and spelling: What speech-language pathologists and teachers need to know. *Language, Speech and Hearing Services in Schools*, 51(4), 939–954.

Nippold, M A and Scott, C M (2010) *Expository Discourse in Children, Adolescents, and Adults: Development and Disorders*. New York: Psychology Press.

Norbury, C F, Gooch, D, Wray, C, Baird, G, Charman, T, Simonoff, E, Vamvakas, G, and Pickles, A (2016) The impact of nonverbal ability on prevalence and clinical presentation of language disorder: evidence from a population study. *Journal of Child Psychology and Psychiatry*, 57(11):1247–1257. https://doi.org/10.1111/jcpp.12573

OECD (2021) *21st-Century Readers: Developing Literacy Skills in a Digital World*. Paris: PISA, OECD Publishing. https://doi.org/10.1787/a83d84cb-en

Perera, K (1984) *Children's Writing and Reading: Analyzing Classroom Language*. Oxford: Blackwell.

Pillinger, C and Vardy, E J (2022) The story so far: A systematic review of the dialogic reading literature. *Journal of Research in Reading*, 45(4): 533–548.

Ruddell, R B, Unrau, N J and McCormick, S (2019) A sociocogntive model of meaning-construction. In Alvermann, D E, Unrau, N J, Sailors, M and Ruddell, R B (eds) *Theoretical Models and Processes of Literacy* (pp 204–232). Seventh edition. New York: Routledge.

Snow, C E (2002) *Reading for Understanding: Toward an R&D Program in Reading Comprehension*. Santa Monica, CA: RAND Corporation. https://www.rand.org/pubs/monograph_reports/MR1465.html

Snow, P C (2016) Elizabeth Usher Memorial Lecture: Language is literacy is language Positioning speech-language pathology in education policy, practice, paradigms and polemics. *International Journal of Speech Language Pathology*, 18(3), 216–228.

Stringer, H, Nicholson, D, and Hope, K (2024) Northumbria Healthcare NHS Foundation Trust - Newcastle University Universal Targeted & Specialist (NNUTS) Framework.

UNESCO (2024) *Global Citizenship Education in a Digital Age: Teacher Guidelines*. Paris: United Nations Educational, Scientific and Cultural Organization. https://doi.org/10.54675/BBSJ1884

Unrau, N J, Alvermann, D E, and Sailors, M (2019) Literacies and their investigation through theories and models. In Alvermann, D E, Unrau, N J, Sailors, M, and Ruddell, R B (eds) *Theoretical Models and Processes of Literacy* (pp 3–34). Seventh edition. New York: Routledge.

Whitehouse, A J O, Line, E A, Watt, H J, and Bishop, D V M (2009) Qualitative aspects of developmental language impairment relate to language and literacy outcome in adulthood. *International Journal of Language & Communication Disorders*, 44(4), 489–510. https://doi.org/10.1080/13682820802708080

Yamaç A, Öztürk E, and Mutlu N (2020) Effect of digital writing instruction with tablets on primary school students' writing performance and writing knowledge. *Computers and Education*, 157: 103981. https://doi.org/10.1016/j.compedu.2020.103981

9 Communication intent and social interaction

Hazel Richards

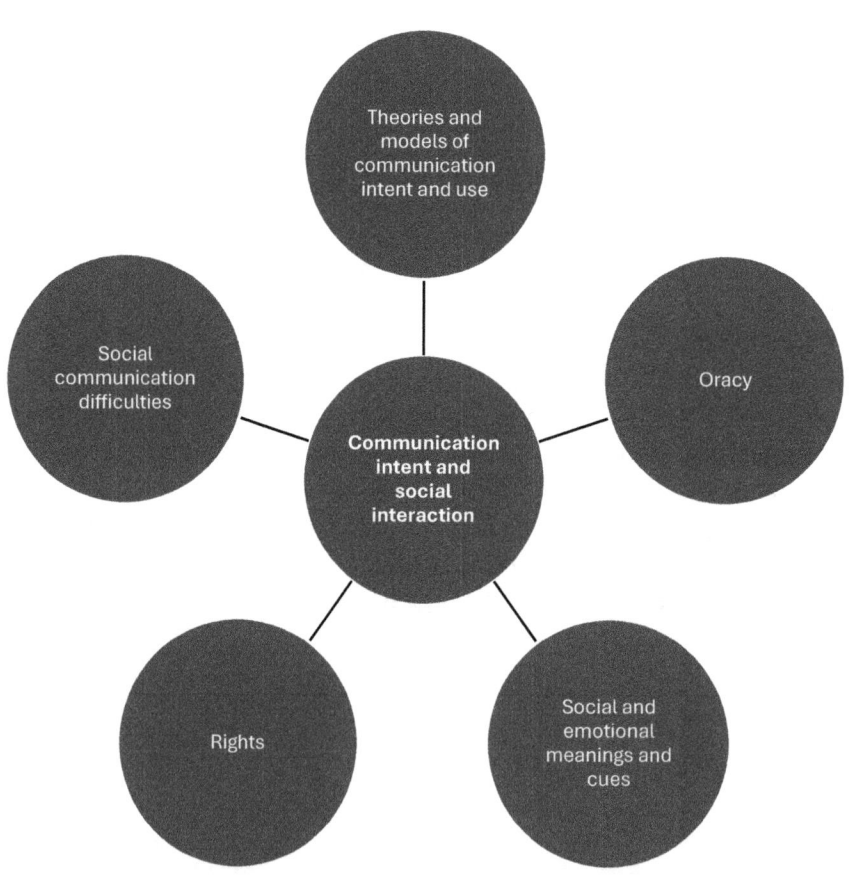

DOI: 10.4324/9781041054986-12

Communication intent and social interaction

🎯 CHAPTER OBJECTIVES

This chapter explores the reasons we communicate. The chapter:

- introduces you to theory and models of communication intent and use;
- explores aspects of oracy;
- considers how we access social and emotional meaning and cues;
- identifies children's rights to communicate and be heard;
- considers when difficulties with communication intent and social interaction are more likely to be present;
- provides guidance for adaptive teaching and signposts to key resources.

🚩 STARTING POINTS

- Why do you talk?
- How does the reason you talk vary between communication partners/settings and your purpose?
- As well as talking, what other ways do you communicate?
- What enhances your desire to communicate?
- What reduces your desire to communicate?

Introduction

Communication is a social activity serving a variety of purposes. It is not just about sending and receiving messages since interaction is involved. Communication skills provide a foundation for social and personal relationships and influence our behaviours, self-regulation and learning. This chapter is therefore concerned with interactions and intentionality (communication use). It is important to consider these, since communication success shapes our motivation to interact and engage further. Also, effective communication requires an understanding of pragmatics. That is, how language is used in context and how social factors influence this. This chapter therefore explores aspects of communication intent and use to help you enhance the social and life chances of the children and young people (CYP) with whom you work.

Theory and models of communication intent and use

Pre-intentional and intentional communication

Newborns vocalise to indicate need and enjoyment, but this is not initially intentional. Rather, intentional communication is built upon developing cognitive understanding (of cause and effect, for example) and social experience. Key stages in this process are detailed in Table 9.1.

Donnellan et al. (2019) found intentionally communicative vocalisations are the best predictors of language and communication development, with transition to intentional communication being a key developmental milestone (Matthews, 2020). Certainly, communication functions, beyond the meeting of basic needs, begin to emerge along with intentionality, with children who show the most initiations for social interaction being found to have the most positive speech, language and communication development outcomes.

Table 9.1 The development of intentional communication

Stage	Child	Caregiver
1. Pre-intentional: reflexive level	Vocalises and cries.	Social significance/meaning is assigned by the caregiver, who responds, creating positive interaction experience.
2. Pre-intentional: reactive level	Vocalisations and cries vary in response to wide range of stimuli, including affect.	As above. Fills in turns, follows line of sight and maps on words, encourages increased variation of sounds.
3. Pre-intentional: pro-active level	Vocalisations increase in range and begin to be tailored to sounds of native language. Behaviours and actions repeated if enjoyed. Child begins to follow carer's line of visual regard.	Reinforces and develops vocalisations through sound play. Interprets vocalisations and movements as intentional as can now extract meaning from child's intonational patterns, voice and facial expression.
4. Intentional: primitive level	Cognitive intention, where child acts on environment to create a specific effect now established. Starts to initiate for social interaction.	Relies heavily on context to understand content and function of the communication. Encodes child's communication. Repeats and encourages anything sounding like speech.
5. Intentional: conventional level	Cognitive intentionality fully established. Signalling through gesture and protowords is recognisable. Meanings conveyed by child, and communicative functions expand rapidly.	Affirms communication by responding to and mapping/expanding message. Conversational turns well established.

Based on Coupe O'Kane and Goldbart, 2016, pp 59–66.

Communication reasons and intent

Money and Thurman's means, reasons and opportunities model (2002) recognises the importance of intentionality and can help identify areas to focus on to develop communication use and effectiveness. The means we communicate includes any method used, including spoken, written, signs and symbols, non-verbal/body language and how we use our voices (for example, volume, intonation, rate and tone) with a total communication approach valuing all means of communication in recognition that this enhances communicative success and so confidence.

Multiple reasons to communicate exist. Children progress from vocalisations that have no obvious communication intent (the pre-intentional stage, see Table 9.1) to increasingly sophisticated functions (Clifford et al., 2010):

Higher-level communicative functions are built upon these earlier communication functions (Figure 9.1) and emerge alongside increasingly abstract thinking. The oracy skills detailed under reasoning (for example, giving reasons to support views and critically examining ideas), audience awareness (taking account of the audience's level of understanding), and rhetorical language (using non-literal or figurative language to convey more abstract meanings through the use of, for example, metaphors, idioms, irony and sarcasm), require knowledge both of commonly held understandings and skilful movement between shared and individually held knowledge.

As children transition into adolescence and beyond, expository discourse and critical thinking increase. Described as the *'language of the curriculum'* (Ward-Lonergan, 2010, p. 242), expository discourse denotes how technical information is conveyed through both written (textbooks and other sources) and spoken (teacher content) means (see Chapter 8). High school teaching and learning requires students to read, analyse and synthesise written and taught information, with assessment being through oral reports and written examinations. Critical thinking, a metacognitive activity which develops during adolescence and beyond, enables individuals to evaluate statements made by advertisers and politicians, distinguish facts from opinions (e.g. in the media), and judge the

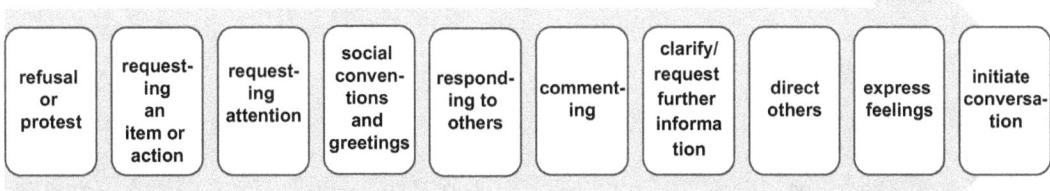

Figure 9.1 Early communication functions (developed from Clifford et al. 2010)

credibility of sources (Nippold et al., 2020). These higher-level communication functions have been linked to better educational and wellbeing outcomes.

We also use language to express choices and preferences – a function that can be harnessed effectively to enable communication about things that are meaningful to the individual (Bloom et al., 2020). Opportunities to communicate can be increased by structuring or manipulating parts of tasks, for example, by leaving a part of the activity/ equipment out so it must be requested; by giving choices rather than just merely handing items to them – e.g. 'do you want an apple or a banana?' and by involving CYP in all decisions that affect them. Opportunities to communicate will also be increased by extending the people, places, times and activities where CYP communicate.

Oracy

The term oracy is used in education to denote speaking and listening skills central *"in the development of the personality and closely related to human happiness and wellbeing"* (Wilkinson, 1970, p. 75), although it has been critiqued as *"a vague term that seems to cover any school activity that involves speaking"* (Teaching Battleground, 2023). Confident and effective communicators become empowered citizens. However, whilst it is stated that it is the job of every classroom teacher, whatever the subject, to develop oracy skills (Rees-Bidder, 2019), teachers' confidence (Dockrell et al., 2017; Mercer and Mannion, 2018) and 'Knowledge About Language' (Jones, 2016, p. 500) can be low, due in part to limited coverage in initial teacher training.

Mapping the four strands (physical, linguistic, cognitive, and social and emotional) of the Oracy Skills Framework (Voice21, 2020) onto the means (how we communicate), reasons (why we communicate) and opportunities (where, when and with whom we communicate) framework (Money and Thurman, 2002) may progress practitioner understanding of areas to target to enhance communication use and effectiveness (Figure 9.2):

Social communication

Communicative competence requires understanding of language use rules since these enable communicators to decide which forms to use in different contexts, and to learn when and how to say something depending on who you are talking to (Bloom and Lahey, 1978). Communication competence is linked to positive outcomes, with adult attention and interpretation playing a key role in validating and developing a CYP's communications. However, practitioners might feel less confident about how to support and develop this.

Bloom and Lahey's (1978) original model separated out content (what we communicate) and form (how we communicate it) from communication use, with the communication context and the agency and intentionality of the CYP contributing to use. Tensions between effort (cognitive processing) and engagement (affect and social interaction) also need to be considered.

Communication intent and social interaction • **129**

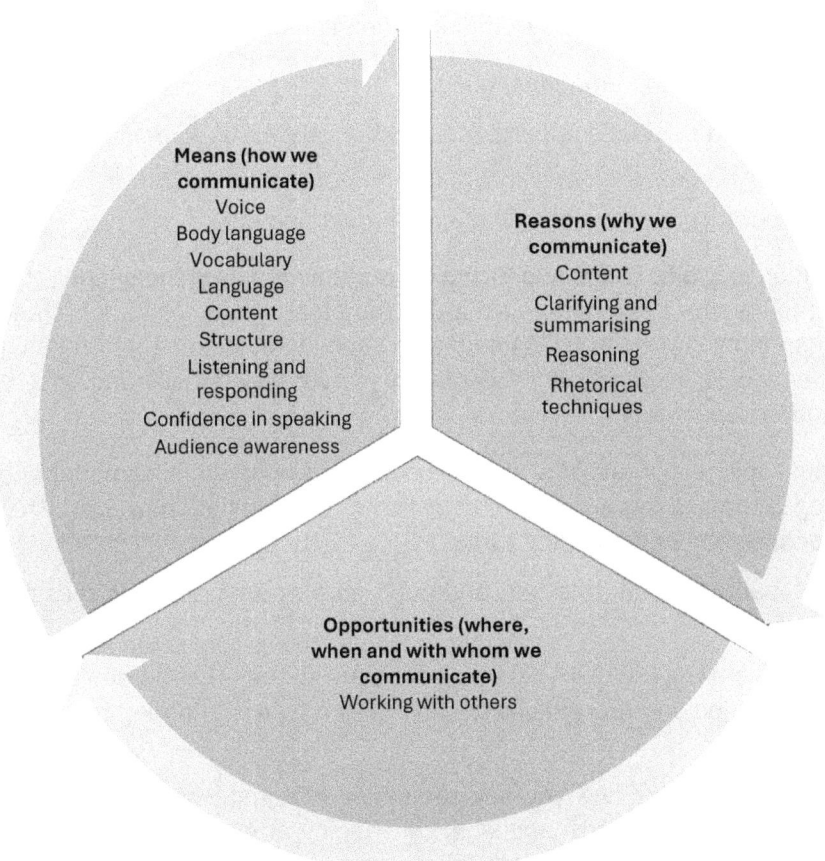

Figure 9.2 *The four strands of oracy mapped onto Money and Thurman's original means, reasons and opportunities model (Money and Thurman, 2002, p. 5)*

ⓘ CRITICAL QUESTIONS

- What are the principle means you use to teach and communicate with your students and how do you supplement these to increase effectiveness?

- What are the main reasons your students communicate in the classroom and around school?

- How might you change aspects of where, when and with whom your students communicate to increase both their need/motivation to communicate and opportunity to do so?

Sociolinguistic rules govern how we pragmatically adapt our language use to meet various situations and environments. Communication competence requires us to:

- apprehend social and emotional cues;
- hold social and semantic understanding which allows us to decipher their meaning, then;
- adapt our own communication to respond appropriately.

Communication is dyadic. Back and forth conversation requires the sender of a message to convey it to the other person in such a way the other person can understand the message and its meaning. Grice (1975) suggested communication cannot take place if participants don't have a common interest (no matter how small) and that successful communication depends on:

- quantity – tailoring messages to a particular listener by thinking about and adapting messages to what your listener already knows or needs to know and by having a balance of speaking and listening turns;
- quality – being truthful, relevant, and polite and by ensuring your message is clear and concise;
- relevance – staying on topic and being sensitive to the other person's contribution to the conversation and recognising what is the wrong or right thing to say in particular contexts;
- manner – considering how you say something (not just what you say), for example, considering tone and body language, by avoiding ambiguous language such as idioms, or by helping your listener to follow when a topic change is occurring.

Social communication challenges are often experienced by autistic people since the social cognitive difficulties in perspective-taking associated with autism mean some communicators find it difficult to understand how their interaction and communication style is perceived by their communication partners. Milton's (2012) double empathy or theory-of-mind problem explains the difference of understanding non-autistic people can experience when interacting with autistic people and vice versa (see 'spotlight on emerging debates' on p. 135). Successful communication therefore requires both semantic understanding (Chapter 7) and the ability to read and adjust to social and emotional meanings and cues.

The right to communicate and be heard

The concepts of voice (as in agency and views) and participation are central to person-centred care, to the United Nations Convention on the Rights of the Child (UNCRC) (Unicef, 1990) and to legislation in England including the Equality Act (2010), the Children and Families Act 2014 and the SEND Code of Practice (DfE and DoH, 2015). Article 12 (UNCRC) details the right of children to express a view, and to have the view given due weight in all matters affecting them. Reviews of implementation of the SEND Code of

Practice reveal variation in the involvement of parents, families and children (Gov.uk, 2023) and the sphere of safeguarding reveals repeated failure to listen to or respond to the voice of CYP. Indeed, practitioner skill influences both how children's voice are accessed (Lundy, 2018) and how the views of CYP are listened, weighted and responded to.

The practice of actively involving children in decision making by supporting them to communicate their wishes should not be conceptualised as an option which is in the gift of the adult, but as a legal imperative which is the right of the child. Supporting our CYP and their families to communicate about and self-identify priorities, results in more favourable responses to interventions and enhanced outcomes (Ofsted, 2019) (see Chapter 12). Suitable methods for eliciting the voices of CYP and families to gain insight into their experiences, strengths and areas they need help with must facilitate both expression and participation (Murphy, 2010; Bloom, et al., 2020). This requires four key elements:

- **representation**, (which requires processes and spaces to be provided that enable CYP to speak for themselves, or to have their position conveyed without adult bias);
- **impact** (how voice is engaged with, responded to and acted upon);
- **judgement** (viewing CYP as capable of making informed decisions, based on them being provided with information and supported to make judgements about issues that concern them); and
- **validity** (CYP's perceptions regarded as valid as, or sometimes more valid than, adult opinions and ideas).

(Jones and Welch, 2018:124)

The challenge for practitioners is to reflect and identify how they are facilitating true voice and participation.

ⓘ CRITICAL QUESTIONS

- Which spaces and tools (means) do you use to support CYP to communicate their wishes?
- What areas of their lives or daily activities do you consult CYP about (reasons)?
- How and when are CYP's perceptions and decisions sought in your practice (opportunities)?
- What gaps and areas to progress tangible changes for your CYP have you identified from answering these questions?

CASE STUDY

Lois – Teaching, learning and communication lead, special school for severe, profound and multiple learning needs

Pupil A is in KS1 and diagnosed with autism and global developmental delay. He is non-verbal and working at approximately 49 months in all developmental areas. When he started in my class, he was occupied with sensory-seeking behaviours such as climbing onto every surface and shuffling small world objects through his fingers or exploring them orally. He expressed himself through facial expressions and vocalisations – primarily to convey enjoyment or discomfort, and struggled to focus and attend on any adult-led activities – attending for around 30 seconds before becoming dysregulated.

In September, our goal was to establish a routine and structure for Pupil A by using a visual timetable and the 'Now and Next' approach. It was also vital to introduce a variety of communication methods (e.g. symbols and signing) and use them in conjunction with verbal communication and to ensure all staff used these consistently throughout the school day, not just in activities, so he had a means to communicate at all times.

As the weeks progressed, Pupil A developed trust in his familiar adults, realising they could meet his needs and were providing consistent responses to his behaviours. Through the use of intensive interaction and interactive games he started to take the adult's hand to what he wanted and tolerated adult interaction for longer periods of time, and he started to make eye contact and smile when the adult copied his actions and vocalisations.

The use of attention autism sessions started to impact Pupil A's ability to focus and attend to adult-led activities and by the end of the academic year, he was able to focus up to stage 2 (sustain attention) almost independently. He would make eye contact and smile and started to show anticipation of what was coming next. All interventions were used with symbols and signs, modelling their use and verbally commenting on what was happening. He progressed from being non-verbal and very insular to showing curiosity and enjoying his interactions with adults, including seeking them out independently and beginning to copy the adults' vocalisations.

Pupil A's good progress is a testament to using a variety of strategies and creating a consistent routine, though I believe his progress could have been even greater. One of the greatest challenges faced was staffing. We had a high turnover of teaching assistants (TA) thus the TA post was often not filled meaning we had to revert to agency staff. This required constant training of staff and enforcing the need to focus on communication.

ⓘ Critical questions

- What changes in staff understanding might be needed to ensure all staff use communication strategies consistently throughout the school day, not just in activities, so ensuring the means to communicate is available to CYP at all times?
- How could consistency of staff and consistent use of strategies have further developed Pupil A's communication?

 SPOTLIGHT ON EMERGING DEBATES

When difficulties with communication use may be more present

Whether we view autism as a disability that can be ameliorated by adapting the surrounding environment (Rieser, 2023), or a difference that is just one of many ways of living life, informs how we respond to and support autistic students. The neurodiversity movement considers how each person's brain develops differently and seeks to de-pathologise autism, one type of neurodivergence and advocates for the rights and interests of individuals with autism. Autism is characterised by communication and interaction differences, which may include challenges initiating and sustaining reciprocal social interaction and social communication (WHO, 2024). We know:

- individuals along the spectrum exhibit a full range of intellectual functioning and language abilities;
- individual presentations can be inherently disabling in some contexts;
- differences in, for example, the perception and processing of sensory input, are a physiological fact (Marco et al., 2011); and
- being able to communicate effectively and understand how verbal and non-verbal communication is affected by intersectional experiences, cultural differences and other factors.

Autistic people are increasingly involved in research to help us understand how they experience and manage the world. Building an appreciation of the challenges and social cognition of individual CYP informs how we support and communicate with them.

Doherty et al.'s (2023) SPACE framework, developed to meet the needs of autistic people in healthcare settings can also be applied in educational settings:

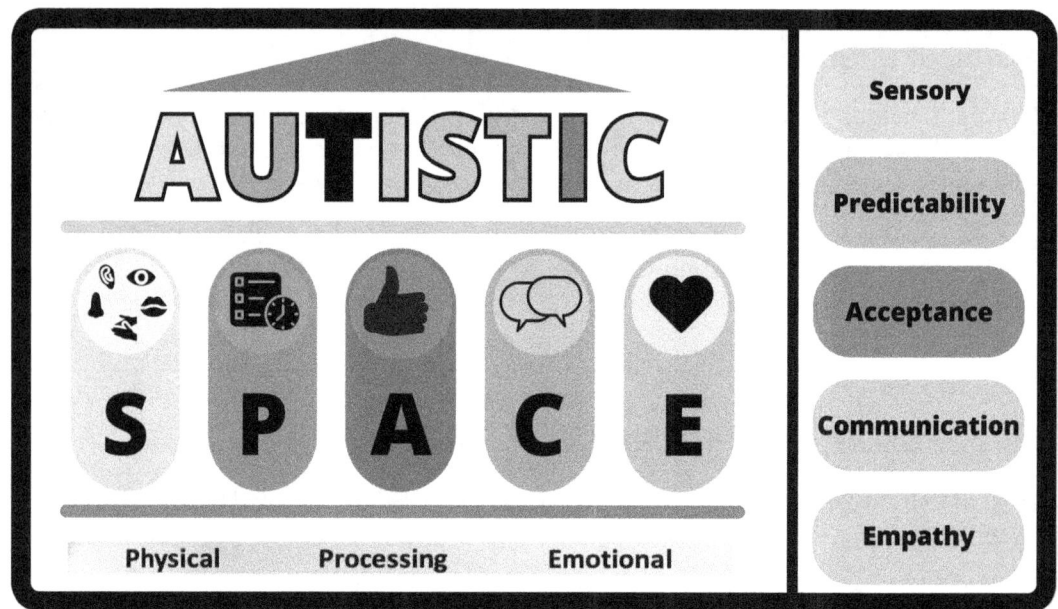

Figure 9.3 *Autistic SPACE (reproduced with kind permission from the authors) Doherty et al.'s (2023)*

The acronym 'SPACE' (Figure 9.3) offers a simple framework of areas to consider and adjust:

- sensory needs (some communicative environments can be overwhelming);
- need for predictability;
- acceptance (of neurodevelopmental differences and by using neurodiverse affirming approaches);
- communication (language use and comprehension is highly variable between individuals and will be suppressed by anxiety and sensory stress, Cummins et al. 2020);
- empathy (including hyper-empathy and/or experiencing or expressing empathy differently).

Autistic individuals can also benefit from adaptations to their physical, processing and emotional spaces, for example, by giving them more time or access to quiet places.

The SCERTS approach (Prizant et al. (2006) and Greenspan Floortime Approach® (Greenspan & Wieder, 2006)) are also worth considering for their focus on social communication and an individualised approach. An individualised approach is also necessary, since how autistic individuals process language varies. Some process phrases in contexts as a whole (known as gestalt language processing, see Chapter 7), whereas others follow more standard language acquisition stages (Hutchins et al., 2024). It is therefore essential to approach the communication and social interaction skills of autistic individuals using person-centred, neurodiversity-affirming approaches that are sensitive and responsive to heterogeneity.

GUIDANCE FOR ADAPTIVE TEACHING

Pupils learn at different rates and require different levels and types of support to succeed. Seeking to understand pupils' differences, including their different levels of communication knowledge and functioning, which are potential barriers to learning, and to respond to these, is therefore an essential part of teaching.

Communicators functioning at a very early level

Assessing the levels of intention (Table 9.1) and communication functions used (Figure 9.1) through interactive activities and using B-squared (see further reading/resources below) will help identify levels of functioning, and next skills to target in your learning outcomes, including how to break down an outcome into smaller steps.

Communicators functioning across the school day

Assessing the means, reasons and opportunities CYP have to communicate during their school day will help you identify and build additional means, reasons and opportunities into your schemes of work/lesson plans and across the school day (not just in activities – see case study). The Autistic SPACE framework will help you to assess aspects of the environment and their impact on communication and learning.

Communication partners make a difference since what others do influences communication (Cummins et al., 2020). The EEF (2021) recommends:

1. Creating a positive and supportive environment for all pupils without exception.
2. Building an ongoing, holistic understanding of your pupils and their needs using the graduated approach of 'assess, plan, do, review'.
3. That good teaching for pupils with SEND is good teaching for all (and so for CYP with speech, language and communication needs). This includes pedagogical strategies, used flexibly in response to the needs of all pupils, with the 'five-a-day' approaches being well-evidenced as beneficial:

- **Teacher instruction** focusing on clear explanations, modelling and frequent checks of understanding;
- **Managing cognitive (and sensory and language) loads** (for example, via clear, tidy classrooms, natural light, labelled drawers, etc.);
- **Scaffolding**, by providing the supports individual pupils need to carry out tasks as autonomously as possible;
- **Flexible grouping**. Complementing high-quality teaching with carefully selected small-group and one-to-one interventions;

→

- Using both **low-tech materials**, for example, using concrete or pictorial supports to convey meaning, and **high-tech materials**, for example, to demonstrate and model and to help pupils learn, practise and record.

Specific resources to develop social communication and interaction include:

- The Talkabout Series (Kelly, A). Based on teaching CYP in groups in school or college, it has resources aimed at different ages from children to teenagers to adults with the aim to develop self-esteem, social and friendship skills. Available at: https://www.winslowresources.com/specific-needs/the-talkabout-series.html (accessed 7 January 2025).
- Language for Behaviour and Emotions (Branagan, A, Cross, M and Parsons, S). Most suitable for Key Stages 2 and 3. Provides a systematic approach to developing: 1) understanding language, 2) emotional literacy skills, 3) inferencing and verbal reasoning skills, 4) narrative skills, 5) social problem-solving. Available at: Language for Behaviour and Emotions: A Practical Guide to Working with (routledge.com; https://www.routledge.com/Language-for-Behaviour-and-Emotions-A-Practical-Guide-to-Working-with-Children-and-Young-People/Branagan-Cross-Parsons/p/book/9780367331832) (accessed 7 January 2025).
- Social Stories (Gray, C). Bespoke personal texts written by authors following a prescribed structure to enable understanding of a particular challenge or social situation. Originally designed for autistic persons, but with wider application. Information available at: Social Stories - Best Practice Resource (middletown-autism.com; https://best-practice.middletownautism.com/approaches-of-intervention/social-stories/) (accessed 7 January 2025).
- Comic Strip Conversations (Gray, C). A visual way to help explore a young person's thoughts and feelings about a situation. Information available at: Social stories and comic strip conversations (autism.org.uk; https://www.autism.org.uk/advice-and-guidance/topics/communication/communication-tools/social-stories-and-comic-strip-coversations) (accessed 7 January 2025).

NB It is not effective to teach these skills through paper-based activities alone, and certainly not 1:1 with an adult. Social interactions occur within live and context - specific situations – so these skills need to be taught within these contexts and in relation to them.

CHAPTER SUMMARY

We do not acquire a language and then learn to communicate with it, rather we learn language via the process of communication. This is because successful communication and social interactions affirm, encourage and stimulate further interactions, leading to progress and development of the speech, language and communication skills that are so integral to teaching and learning and to pupil outcomes and well-being. This chapter therefore considered key aspects of this and signposted valuable resources to help you intentionally develop communication intent and social interaction skills in the CYP you work with.

 Further reading/resources

Talking Mats | Improving communication, improving lives (https://www.talkingmats.com/)

- Talking Mats increase the capacity of people with communication difficulties to think about and communicate effectively about things that matter to them. They can be adapted for any curriculum or life area.

B-Squared (2023) *Autism Progress: supporting autistic students to achieve Handbook. An Introduction and Guide to Using the Autism Progress Profiling Tool.* Available at: Autism Progress Handbook (bsquared.co.uk; https://www.bsquared.co.uk/wp-content/uploads/2021/08/Autism-Progress-Handbook.pdf) (accessed 7 January 2025).

- The 17 level descriptors (for communication, social interaction, flexibility of though and emotional regulation) support both assessment and identification of learning objectives.

 References

Attention Autism (n.d.) Attention Autism Ltd – Support Services for Autism (accessed 18 March 2025).

Bloom, A, Critten, S, Johnson, H, and Wood, C (2020) A critical review of methods for eliciting voice from children with speech, language and communication needs. *Journal of Research in Special Educational Needs*, 20(4): 308–320.

Bloom, L and Lahey, M (1978) *Language Development and Language Disorders*. New York: Wiley.

B-Squared (2023) *Autism Progress: supporting autistic students to achieve Handbook. An Introduction and Guide to Using the Autism Progress Profiling Tool.* Available at: Autism Progress Handbook (bsquared.co.uk; https://www.bsquared.co.uk/wp-content/uploads/2021/08/Autism-Progress-Handbook.pdf) (accessed 18 March 2025).

Clifford, S, Hudry, K, Brown, L, Pasco, G and Charman T (2010) The Modified Classroom Observation Schedule to Measure Intentional Communication (M-COSMIC): Evaluation of reliability and validity. *Research in Autism Spectrum* Disorders, 4(3): 509–525.

Coupe O'Kane, J and Goldbart, J (2016) *Communication before Speech: Development and Assessment*. 2nd ed. Abingdon: Routledge.

Cummins, C, Pellicano, E and Crane, L (2020) Autistic adults' views of their communication skills and needs. *International Journal of Language and Communication Disorders*, 55(5): 678–689

DfE and DoH (Department for Education and Department of Health) (2015) *Special educational needs and disability code of practice: 0 to 25 years*. Available at: https://www.gov.uk/government/publications/send-code-of-practice-0-to-25 (accessed 18 March 2025).

Dockrell, J, Howell, P, Leung, D, and Fugard, A (2017) Children with speech language and communication needs in England: Challenges for practice. *Frontier Education*, 2(35): 1–14.

Doherty, M, McCowan, S, and Shaw, S C (2023) Autistic SPACE: A novel framework for meeting the needs of autistic people in healthcare settings. *British Journal of Hospital Medicine*, 84(4): 1–9.

Donnellan, E, Bannard, C, McGillion, M L, Slocombe, A E, and Matthews, D (2019) Infants' intentionally communicative vocalizations elicit responses from caregivers and are the best predictors of the transition to language: A longitudinal investigation of infants' vocalizations, gestures and word production. *Developmental Science* 23(1) https://doi.org/10.1111/desc.12843

EEF (Educational Endowment Foundation) (2021) *Special Educational Needs in Mainstream Schools: Create a positive learning environment for pupils with SEN*. Available at: https://educationendowmentfoundation.org.uk/education-evidence/guidance-reports/send (accessed 18 March 2025).

Equality Act (2010). Available at https://www.legislation.gov.uk/ukpga/2010/15/contents (accessed 18 March 2025).

Gov.uk (2023) *SEND and alternative provision improvement plan*. Available at: SEND and alternative provision improvement plan - GOV.UK (www.gov.uk; https://www.gov.uk/government/publications/send-and-alternative-provision-improvement-plan) (accessed 18 March 2025).

Greenspan, S I and Wieder S (2006) *Engaging Autism: Using the Floortime Approach to Help Children Relate, Communicate, and Think*. Da Capo Lifelong.

Grice, H P (1975) Logic and conversation. In Cole, P and Morgan, J (eds) *Syntax and Semantics: Speech Arts*. New York: Academic Press, pp. 41–58. Available at: Grice-Logic_and_Conversation.pdf (partiallyexaminedlife.com; https://partiallyexaminedlife.com/wp-content/uploads/Grice-Logic_and_Conversation.pdf) (accessed 18 March 2025).

Hutchins, T L, Knox, S E, and Fletcher, E C (2024) Natural language acquisition and gestalt language processing: A critical analysis of their application to autism and speech language therapy. *Autism and Developmental Language Impairments*, 9, 1–9. https://doi.org/10.1177/23969415241249944

Jones, D (2016) Talking about talk: Reviewing oracy in English primary education. *Early Child Development and Care*, 187(3–4): 498–508. https://doi.org/10.1080/03004430.2016.1211125

Jones, P and Welch, S (2018) *Rethinking Children's Rights: Attitudes in Contemporary Society*. London: Bloomsbury Publishing.

Lundy, L (2018) In defence of tokenism? Implementing children's right to participate in collective decision-making. *Childhood*, 25(3): 340–354.

Marco, E J, Hinkley, L B N, Hill, S S, and Nagarajan, S S (2011) Sensory processing in autism: A review of neurophysiologic findings. *Pediatric Research*, 69(5 Pt 2): 48R–54R.

Matthews, D (2020) Learning to communicate in infancy. In Rowland, C F, Theakston, A F, Ambridge, B, and Twomey, K E *Current Perspectives on Child Language Acquisition*. Philadelphia: John Benjamins.

Mercer, N M and Mannion, J (2018) *Oracy across the Welsh Curriculum. A Research-Based Review: Key Principles and Recommendations for Teachers*. Oracy Cambridge report for the Welsh Government. Available at: Oracy-across-the-Welsh-curriculum-July-2018.pdf (oracycambridge.org; https://oracycambridge.org/wp-content/uploads/2018/07/Oracy-across-the-Welsh-curriculum-July-2018.pdf) (accessed 18 March 2025).

Milton, D (2012) On the ontological status of autism: The 'double empathy problem'. *Disability and Society*, 27(6): 883–887.

Money, D and Thurman, S (2002) Towards a model of inclusive communication. *Speech and Language Therapy in Practice*. Autumn, 4–6. Available at: Inclusive Communication - Coming Soon Near You? | Download Free PDF | Disability | Inclusion (Education) (scribd.com) (accessed 18 March 2025).

Murphy, J (2010) *Talking Mats: a study of communication difficulties and the feasibility and effectiveness of a low-tech communication framework*. Available at: Talking Mats: A Study of Communication Difficulties and the Feasibility and Effectiveness of a Low-Tech Communication Framework | Request PDF (researchgate.net; https://www.researchgate.net/publication/254880638_Talking_Mats_A_Study_of_Communication_Difficulties_and_the_Feasibility_and_Effectiveness_of_a_Low-Tech_Communication_Framework) (accessed 18 March 2025).

Nippold, A, LaFavre, S, and Shinham, K (2020) How Adolescents Interpret the Moral Messages of Fables: Examining the Development of Critical Thinking. *Journal of Speech, Language, and Hearing Research*, 63(4): 1212–1226.

OFSTED (2019) Education Inspection Framework: Overview of Research, January 2019. No:180045. Office for Standards in Education, Children's Services and Skills. Available at: Research for education inspection framework (publishing.service.gov.uk; https://assets.publishing.service.gov.uk/media/6034be17d3bf7f265dbbe2ef/Research_for_EIF_framework_updated_references_22_Feb_2021.pdf) (accessed 18 March 2025).

Prizant, B, Wetherby, A, Rubin, E, Laurent, A, and Rydell, P (2006) *The SCERTS Model: A Comprehensive Educational Approach to Children with Autistic Spectrum Disorders*. Baltimonre, MD: Paul Brookes Publishing.

Rees-Bidder, H (2019) *What is Oracy and Why Does It Matter?* Cambridge: Cambridge Assessment. Available at: What is oracy and why does it matter? | Cambridge Assessment (https://www.cambridgeassessment.org.uk/blogs/what-is-oracy-and-why-does-it-matter/) (accessed 18 March 2025).

Rieser, R (2023) Disability equality: The last civil right? In Cole, M. (ed) (2nd edition) *Education, Equality and Human Rights: Issues of Gender, 'Race', Sexuality, Disability and Social Class*. Abingdon: Routledge, pp. 175–215.

Teaching Battleground (2023) Oracy and the EEF. Part 1. Available at: Oracy and the EEF. Part 1 | Scenes From The Battleground (wordpress.com; https://teachingbattleground.wordpress.com/2023/09/21/oracy-and-the-eef-part-1/) (accessed 18 March 2025).

Unicef (United Nations Convention of the Rights of the Child (UNCRC) (1990). Available at: http://www.unicef.org.uk/wp-content/uploads/2010/05/UNCRC_united_nations_convention_on_the_rights_of_the_child.pdf (accessed 18 March 2025).

Voice21 (2020) *The Oracy Skills Framework*. Available at: https://www.educ.cam.ac.uk/research/programmes/oracytoolkit/oracyskillsframework/Oracy%20Skills%20Framework%202020.pdf (accessed 18 March 2025).

Ward-Lonergan, J M (2010) Expository discourse intervention: Helping school-age children and adolescents with language disorders master the language of the curriculum. Chapter 10 in Nippold, M. A. and Scott, C. M. (eds) *Expository Discourse in Children, Adolescents, and Adults: Development and Disorders*. Hove: Psychology Press, (pp. 242–284). https://doi.org/10.4324/9780203848821

WHO (2024) International Classification of Diseases-11. Available at: ICD-11 for Mortality and Morbidity Statistics (who.int) (accessed 18 March 2025).

Wilkinson, A (1970) The concept of oracy. *The English Journal*, 59(1): 71–77.

10 Enabling communication for children who stammer

Aaron Emmett

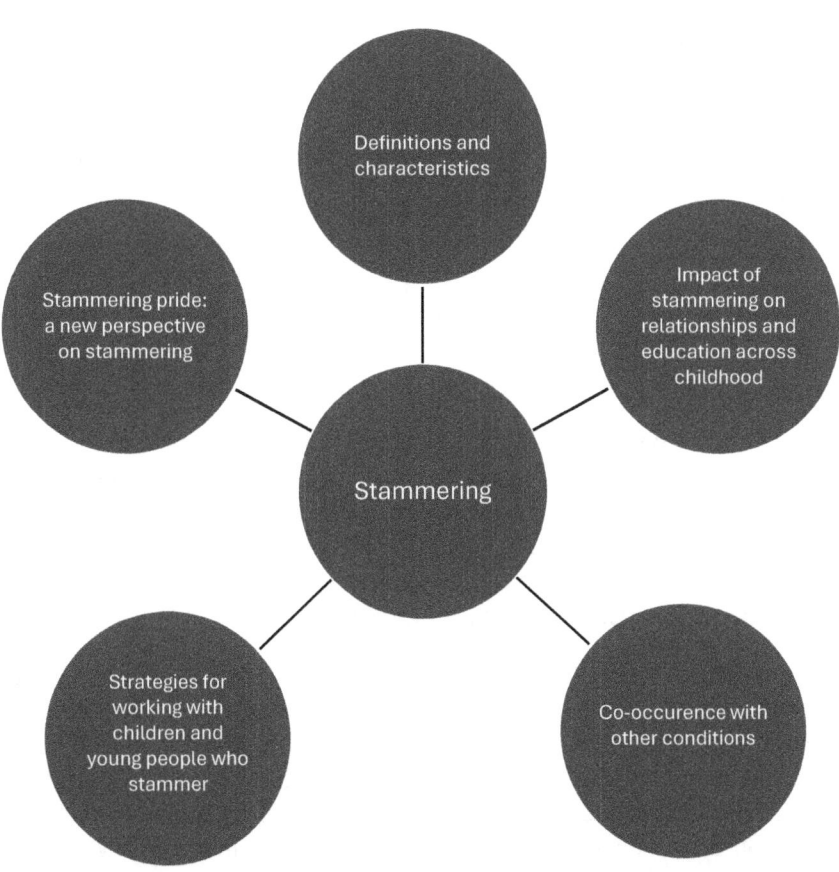

DOI: 10.4324/9781041054986-13

> ### CHAPTER OBJECTIVES
>
> This chapter explores the nature of stammering and its impact on children and young people. The chapter:
>
> - outlines the key terminology around stammering;
> - considers the characteristics of stammering that the listener may see and hear, and those that are internally experienced by the person who stammers;
> - identifies some of the impacts on stammering and how these are relevant to education settings;
> - suggests strategies for working with children and young people who stammer to access learning with confidence.

Introduction

Stammering is a communication difference characterised by an interruption in the flow of speech. This can manifest in different ways, including:

- repetition of sounds or whole words e.g. 'h-h-he got the ball' or 'he-he-he got the ball';
- prolongation or 'stretching out' sounds e.g. 'Sssssstop that!';
- blocking, where speech gets stuck and no sound is produced.

Alongside the speech characteristics, people who stammer may also experience 'secondary' or 'concomitant' behaviours – bodily movements or signs of tension that occur alongside the stammer. There are multiple types of secondary behaviours which include but are not limited to: tension in the face, tapping feet and clenching fists. Secondary behaviours are not always present in people who stammer and some individuals may not experience them consistently every time they stammer.

In the UK, stammering is the preferred term, but stuttering may also be used to describe the same phenomenon and is becoming more common. These terms are interchangeable – there is no difference between stammering and stuttering. In medical terms, stammering is sometimes known as 'dysfluency'. We should use the term that the person who stammers/stutters prefers. To avoid confusion, stammering will be used throughout this chapter. It is worth noting that every talker will experience some instances where they are not completely fluent, for example, when they are tired or nervous, but this is distinct from stammering in its frequency, characteristics and impact.

Estimates vary but research suggests that around 1% of the population stammer (Lee, 2023). This means that in the United Kingdom, there are potentially nearly 700,000 individuals who stammer.

> **🏁 STARTING POINTS**
>
> - Can you think of any children or young people you have worked with who stammer?
> - What do you feel you already know about stammering?
> - Can you think of any time you have seen stammering portrayed, e.g. on TV or in film?

What causes stammering?

Stammering is a complicated phenomenon and as technology advances, so too does our understanding of how and why stammering occurs. Stammering can be considered 'multi-factorial' in that there are several elements which contribute to an individual's experience of their stammer.

Thanks to studies that investigate the differences in brain structures and functions, we know that the parts of the brain responsible for speech production work slightly differently for people who stammer compared to people who do not. There is evidence to suggest that for people who stammer, the part of the brain that starts speech muscles moving works typically, but the part of the brain that stops speech movement behaves differently (Chang and Guenther, 2020). This leads to the repetitive speech patterns that characterise stammering. Whilst there is strong support for a neurological (brain-based) element to stammering, further research is needed to explain exactly what is occurring.

There is also strong evidence for a genetic influence to stammering. Sixty per cent of people who stammer have a close relative who also stammers, for example, a father or grandfather (Darmody et al., 2022). This would suggest that some element of stammering can be inherited from our parents.

Whilst we know that stammering is not caused by an individual's demeanour, personality or mental state, there is evidence to suggest that people who stammer will stammer more when they are nervous, excited, or experiencing 'bigger' emotions (Tichenor and Yaruss, 2021). For example, families often report that their child stammers more frequently around the build-up to the Christmas period because of excitement and anticipation.

Finally, there are instances where stammering occurs from a neurogenic cause – where there is damage to brain, e.g. from a head injury or a psychogenic cause – where stammering occurs because of a psychological event such as trauma (Binder et al., 2012; Junuzovic-Zunic et al., 2021). These types of stammering are rare, however, and most cases of stammering can be considered developmental – they begin in early childhood without a triggering event.

Covert stammering

Stammering can be an intensely difficult and challenging experience for an individual. In some cases, the person who stammers may attempt to use several ways of hiding or masking their stammer (Gattie et al., 2024). These can include:

- Avoiding or replacing words they feel they might stammer on;
- Trying to make a moment of stammering appear like something else is happening;
- Rehearsing speech ahead of time to try to anticipate stammering;
- Avoiding speaking situations entirely.

Covert stammering can be very difficult to identify, and people who covertly stammer can be very adept at hiding their stammer in certain situations. It is important not to make assumptions about children and young people's communication; you may, for example, find a parent or carer reporting that their child stammers at home but this is never noticed at school.

The feeling of needing to hide a stammer is likely in part due to public perceptions of stammering and a fear of negative reactions from listeners. The myths and misconceptions surrounding stammering are numerous and pervasive across society, and as such it is no surprise that some of these beliefs are taken on by people who stammer and internalised, leading to a detrimental impact on their wellbeing.

> ⑦ **CRITICAL QUESTION**
>
> Consider some of the below myths and the realities that refute them; do they match anything you might have thought when you think of stammering?
>
> - *People stammer because they are shy, nervous or lack confidence* – Stammering is caused by physiological differences in the brain, not by nerves. People who stammer may stammer more when they feel anxious, but anxiety does not cause stammering.
> - *People who stammer are less intelligent than their non-stammering peers* – Stammering has no connection to intelligence or academic ability, and people who stammer will have a range of capabilities as do their non-stammering peers.
> - *Stammering is caused by the parents' or carers' actions or parenting style* – The way a child is raised has no bearing on whether they stammer or not. Actions by parents, carers or other adults around the child can have an impact on how the child views their stammer, however.
> - *Stammering is caused by raising a child with more than one language* – Stammering occurs across every language and culture and there is no evidence to suggest raising a child multi-lingual contributes to developing stammering.

Impact of stammering

Outside the direct speech differences that a person who stammers experiences, stammering can affect an individual in several ways. Children and young people who stammer are more vulnerable to mental health difficulties such as anxiety (Bernard et al., 2022) and negative self-views, such as feelings of shame, low self-esteem, and lack of confidence (Erickson and Block, 2013). Perhaps unsurprisingly, feelings of embarrassment and frustration are common, and these can develop and compound throughout childhood and into adolescence and beyond (Eggers et al., 2021).

A common analogy for the experience of a person who stammers is an iceberg (Sheehan, 1970). The part of the iceberg that is visible above the water represents the features of stammering we can see and hear, the speech differences and secondary behaviours like visible tension. Below the surface of the water is the base of the iceberg which represents the invisible features, the thoughts and feelings of shame, isolation, embarrassment and frustration. It is important to consider both the visible and invisible features of stammering. A representation of this can be seen in Figure 10.1.

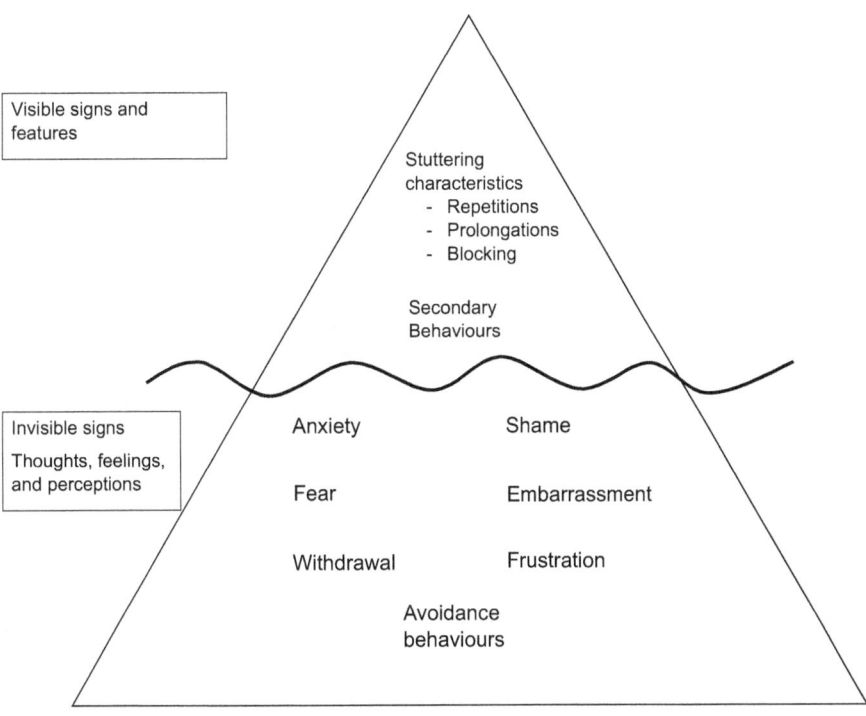

Figure 10.1 *The stammering iceberg analogy*

Stammering and other types of special educational needs

Stammering can affect any individual regardless of their age, gender or background. However, some populations are more likely to stammer than others. Children with neurodevelopmental conditions such as autistic children, children with ADHD or a learning disability, are more likely to stammer compared to their neurotypical peers (Briley and Ellis, 2018). Stammering can also co-occur with other types of speech, language, and communication need such as Speech Sound Disorder (Unicomb et al., 2020). The individual should be considered holistically when making decisions about the types of support they require, giving attention to all areas of need (see Chapters 6 and 9).

 SPOTLIGHT ON NEW DEBATES AND DEVELOPMENTS

The social model of disability suggests that disability is mainly due to systemic barriers, social exclusion and widely held societal perspectives that stop disabled people from being able to fully participate in society. The relevance of this for people who stammer has been elaborated in recent years by academics and the stammering community (Constantino et al., 2022). We have already discussed the stigma and misconceptions that surround stammering which has a huge impact on the experiences of people who stammer. It is important to consider that society holds fluent speech in high regard as a mark of competence in communication. This leads to a perception that stammering is wrong, disordered or generally undesirable. We can see how deeply this pervades the public consciousness by considering the portrayal of people who stammer in the media – characters who stammer are often considered weak, anxious, cowardly, or even presented for comedic effect (Johnson, 2008).

Part of working with people who stammer, as people who do not stammer, is about challenging our perceptions of stammering and fluency and interrogating why we value fluency so highly. There is no evidence to suggest that stammering is linked to lower intelligence, or a reduced capacity to communicate. Indeed, there are many people who stammer who successfully live lives where communication is critical, e.g. in the workplace. There is a drive to acknowledge stammering as a difference, rather than taking the view that it is a deficit – which has been the traditionally held and medically driven view of the past.

The neurodiversity movement is rightly challenging notions of difference vs deficit in other areas, as mentioned in Chapter 9. This paradigm shift is very relevant to stammering and parallels it in many ways – *can society move to a place where stammering is considered simply a different way of communicating, rather than a defective or lesser one* (Sisskin, 2023)? It is therefore incumbent on those working with children and young people who stammer to be aware of these conversations and not perpetuate the notion that stammering is somehow inherently 'bad' or 'wrong'.

Instead, can we support these people by giving them space to communicate authentically and without fear of judgement?

With the discussion of oracy in mind from Chapters 1 and 9, it is important to consider how stammering might intersect with this (Berquez et al., 2011). We must be very careful not to equate fluency with effective communication – they are separate entities. This is relevant to teaching practices and our assessment of pupils. Consider, for example, the way speaking exams and assessments are used to measure pupils' understanding of a subject. We must not include fluency as an indicator of success or we are setting people who stammer up to fail from the start. We also need to very careful of how we are using terminology, e.g. by being very clear on the differences between fluent speech and fluency from a language learning perspective.

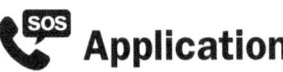

Application

The needs of any individual who stammers are as unique as the individual themselves. With this in mind, the following is a starting point for supports for children and young people who stammer. It is recommended that for any child or young person that stammers, a referral is made to local speech and language therapy services alongside the implementation of these strategies.

The consideration of support for pupils who stammer is not only an ethical and educational one, but a legal one, as stammering is considered to be a disability under the purposes of the Equality Act (2010). Further recommendations for making reasonable adjustments in line with this legislation can be found through STAMMA, signposted in the resources at the end of the chapter.

GUIDANCE FOR ADAPTIVE TEACHING

- **Give the speaker time to finish what they are saying**. It is important not to interrupt a person who stammers before they are finished. Imagine the frustration you might feel if you were interrupted before you had completed what you were saying.

- **Do not try to anticipate what the speaker might be trying to say when they stammer**. Attempting to fill in words or complete a sentence can communicate that we do not value what a person has to say, or that we value them saying it quickly more than the content.

- **Do not encourage the speaker to 'slow down' 'take a breath' or 'stop and start again'**. These suggestions are often well meaning, but they are not usually useful for the person who stammers to hear and can exacerbate the stress in the moment of stammering. It can be hard to watch someone struggle and avoid the temptation to 'rescue' them, but it is important they are given the opportunity to finish what they are saying.
- **Do not look away when the speaker stammers**. If you feel uncomfortable when someone stammers, it is important not to show this to the speaker as this can make them feel uncomfortable in turn. Maintain normal eye contact and show you are listening to what they are saying.
- **If you notice that the speaker is really struggling, it's fine to acknowledge this and assure them they can take as much time as they need**. People who stammer know they are stammering; if it looks particularly effortful, it is ok to give reassurance that you will give them the time they need.

For younger children who stammer, it is important to consider their awareness of their stammer – very young children might not be aware their speech sounds different to their peers. With this in mind:

- **Do not be the first person to raise their stammer with a young child**. Instead, it is more helpful to follow the strategies above and let them know through these that you are listening to what they have to say.
- **Discuss their stammer with their parents or carers and use the language they use if they have spoken to their child about stammering**. When communicating about a complex topic like stammering, families will often have their own vocabulary and we should take this lead and emulate them. This might be, for example, 'bumpy talking' or 'getting stuck'.
- **Give specific praise around all of their activities, not just communication**. Specific praise allows children to recognise what their strengths are. You might want to follow a format of 'you did... and that was' e.g. 'you shared your toys with Billy, that was very kind of you'. There may be times when you do want to praise the young child's communication, so again, be specific: 'I could tell that was a bit tricky to say, but you kept going and I'm really glad you did'.

For older children and teenagers/young adults, it is important that we speak to them and get their views on what is helpful. As the young person gets older, they may have their own ideas about what others do that helps when they stammer. You might like to suggest some of the following strategies if they find it difficult to articulate what would be helpful:

- **Make adjustments to the register**. Answering the register can be a daily stressful occurrence for people who stammer, particularly if their name appears later in the list and there is more time for anxiety around speaking to build. There may be particular difficulties with the sounds in the register response like 'y' in 'yes sir' or the 'h' in 'here miss'. Suggest giving the option to answer in a different way that is easier for the individual. This should be applied to everyone on the register so that it does not single out the young person who stammers.

- **Consider activities where reading aloud is necessary**. If it is required that the young person read aloud in English, for example, consider suggesting that they may want to go first so there is less time to worry about their turn coming up or making it very clear which order the reading will go in so they are able to prepare for their turn.

- **Speak to the young person about contributing to class discussions**. This might include preparing them for being asked a question, or picking them first if they raise their hand to contribute. This can help to minimise the panic of waiting to know if they will be called on to give an answer.

Ultimately, it is important these are implemented in discussion with the young person so they feel in control of their participation.

CASE STUDY

Charlotte, specialist teacher of cognition and learning including speech and language at a universal and targeted level for a local authority, mainstream secondary school setting

As part of a pupil one-to-one assessment as directed by a school I support, I met Paul, a Year 9 pupil. The school were concerned about his learning and progress. It was reported by the school that he was born prematurely and had a stammer which had been previously supported by NHS Speech and Language, however, this support had stopped quite a while ago as his parent thought that the stammer was not impacting on her son and his learning. She wanted him to achieve well and succeed in his future.

It soon became clear that his stammer was still a difficulty when he began to try to express and share his views with me becoming frustrated and visibly upset. He perceived it quite negatively and shared that he wanted it to go away as it affected his life both at home and school. Each interaction with Paul took much longer as he required extra time and space to speak and to find the words he wanted to use. Therefore, it was apparent that he would very much struggle to keep up with the pace of learning in his lessons. I had previously received training and watched programmes on the television around stammering so understood that the pressure for Paul to respond had to be minimised to support his communication.

However, as the assessment continued, Paul shared that he had developed some of his own strategies to cope with the demands of his stutter. He was observed to count off the words as he spoke to try and keep some fluency to what he wanted to say. He also spelt out words aloud or just wrote down what he wanted to say, especially as he became tired with the effort needed. This displayed what problem-solving strengths he had that should be celebrated and used.

Following assessment, in my written report to the school, I recommended that a rereferral to speech and language was urgently required and highlighted that Paul needed access to a much slower pace of learning. He had to be allowed to use his strategies and alternative ways to communicate in his lessons. The school's special educational needs coordinator also shared my report and its findings with his parent. Therefore, on hearing from an outside professional and agreeing with the findings, happily consented to the referral needed back to speech and language therapy for professional support and began to understand her son better, thus alleviating the pressure and expectations from home. I am hoping that Paul's weaknesses and strengths will now be better recognised and that he feels heard and his strengths can be commended so his self-esteem grows especially as he enters Key Stage 4.

Critical questions

- How might changing the environment around Paul help him use strategies – or allow him to need them less often?
- Can you identify where some of the features of Paul's case would go on the stammering iceberg?
- What do you need to work in a collaborative way, like Charlotte did, to involve everybody and let the pupil inform their support?

CHAPTER SUMMARY

The experiences of children and young people who stammer are varied, and they are made more complicated by society's perceptions and misconceptions. It is essential that we carefully consider how best to provide a safe and nurturing environment for them, with input from the individuals and their families. Creating these spaces will ensure that they can feel truly heard for what they have to say, not

Further reading/resources

www.stamma.org

- The official website for the British Stammering Association containing information about stammering for children, young people, families and education staff and resources on making reasonable adjustments.

www.actionforstammeringchildren.org

- A charity that supports children and families of children who stammer. They provide advice, campaign for policy change and fund research into stammering. Their Stambassadors campaign features several adults who stammer talking about their experiences of employment.

 References

Bernard, R, Hofslundsengen, H, and Frazier Norbury, C, (2022) Anxiety and depression symptoms in children and adolescents who stutter: A systematic review and meta-analysis. *Journal of Speech, Language, and Hearing Research*, 65(2): 624–644.

Berquez, A E, Cook, F M, Millard, S K, and Jarvis, E (2011) The stammering information programme: A Delphi study. *Journal of Fluency Disorders*, 36(3): 206–221.

Binder, L M, Spector, J, and Youngjohn, J R (2012) Psychogenic stuttering and other acquired nonorganic speech and language abnormalities. *Archives of Clinical Neuropsychology*, 27(5): 557–568.

Briley, P M, and Ellis Jr, C (2018) The coexistence of disabling conditions in children who stutter: Evidence from the National Health Interview Survey. *Journal of Speech, Language, and Hearing Research*, 61(12): 2895–2905.

Chang, S E and Guenther, F H (2020) Involvement of the cortico-basal ganglia-thalamo-cortical loop in developmental stuttering. *Frontiers in Psychology*, 10: 3088.

Constantino, C, Campbell, P, and Simpson, S (2022) Stuttering and the social model. *Journal of Communication Disorders*, 96: 106200.

Darmody, T, O'Brian, S, Rogers, K, Onslow, M, Jacobs, C, McEwen, A, Lowe, R, Packman, A, and Menzies, R (2022) Stuttering, family history and counselling: A contemporary database. *Journal of fluency disorders*, 73: 105925.

Eggers, K, Millard, S, and Kelman, E (2021) Temperament and the impact of stuttering in children aged 8–14 years. *Journal of Speech, Language, and Hearing Research*, 64(2): 417–432.

Erickson, S and Block, S (2013) The social and communication impact of stuttering on adolescents and their families. *Journal of Fluency Disorders*, 38(4): 311–324.

Gattie, M, Lieven, E, and Kluk, K (2024) Adult stuttering prevalence II: Recalculation, subgrouping and estimate of stuttering community engagement. *Journal of Fluency Disorders*, 83: 106086.

Johnson, J K, (2008) The visualization of the twisted tongue: Portrayals of stuttering in film, television, and comic books. *Journal of Popular Culture*, 41(2), p. 245.

Junuzovic-Zunic, L, Sinanovic, O, and Majic, B (2021) Neurogenic stuttering: Etiology, symptomatology, and treatment. *Medical Archives*, 75(6): 456.

Lee, K (2023) Meta-analysis of stuttering prevalence and incidence. *Communication Sciences & Disorders*, 28(3): 631–642.

Sheehan, J G (1970) *Stuttering: Research and Therapy*. New York: Harper & Row.

Sisskin, V (2023) Disfluency-affirming therapy for young people who stutter: Unpacking ableism in the therapy room. *Language, Speech, and Hearing Services in Schools*, 54(1): 114–119.

The Equality Act (2010) United Kingdom Public General Acts, 2010 c. 15. Available at: https://www.legislation.gov.uk/ukpga/2010/15/contents (Accessed: 23rd of January 2025).

Tichenor, S E and Yaruss, J S (2021) Variability of stuttering: Behavior and impact. *American Journal of Speech-Language Pathology*, 30(1): 75–88.

Unicomb, R, Kefalianos, E, Reilly, S, Cook, F, and Morgan, A (2020) Prevalence and features of comorbid stuttering and speech sound disorder at age 4 years. *Journal of communication disorders*, 84: 105976.

11 Supporting the communication of children and young people with social, emotional and mental health (SEMH) needs

Claire Westwood and Teri Oakshott-Marston

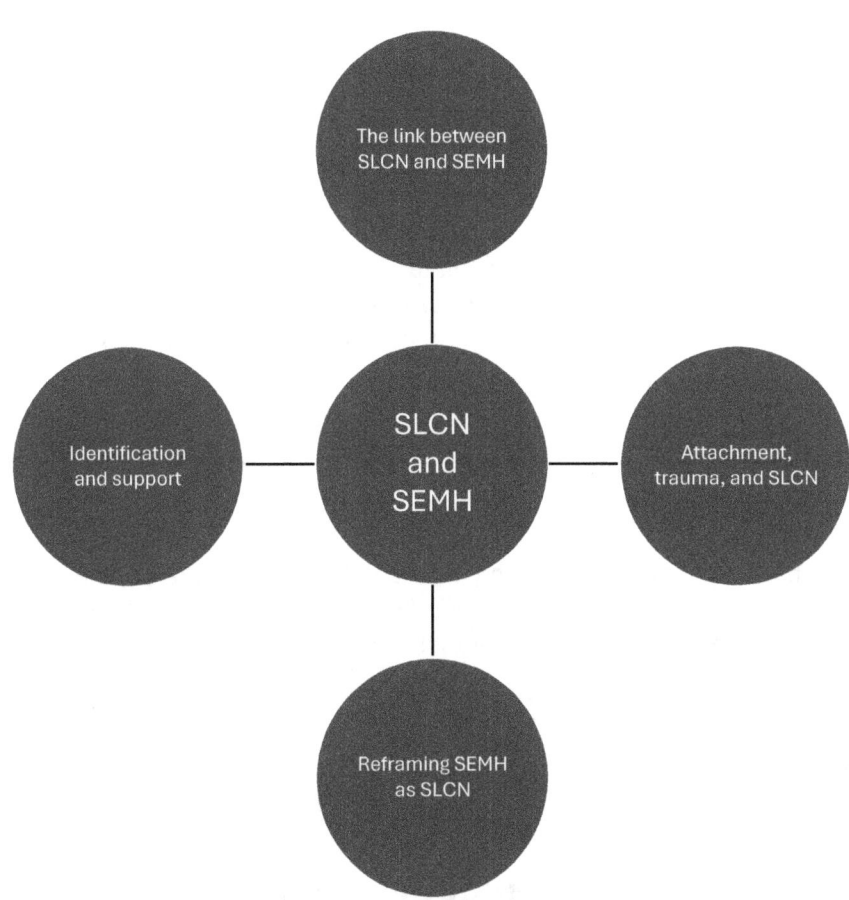

🎯 CHAPTER OBJECTIVES

This chapter explores how social emotional and mental health needs (SEMH) can be related to, often undiagnosed, speech, language and communication needs (SLCN). It aims to:

- provide an overview of how SEMH and SLCN are linked, including relationships to attachment and trauma;
- enable you to reflect upon your experiences of supporting learners with these needs and ask critical questions to extend your practice further;
- discuss a range of real-life case examples to demonstrate children and young people's experiences; and
- provide practical strategies to assist you to identity and support SLCN in learners with SEMH.

Introduction

SEMH is now the second most common category of Special Educational Needs and Disabilities (SEND) in schools, with 24% having SEMH as their primary need (Department for Education, 2024). SEMH is a broad range of experiences that encompasses internalising behaviours e.g. 'becoming withdrawn and isolated' as well as externalising difficulties such as 'challenging, disruptive or disturbing behaviour' (SEND Code of Practice, 2015). These learners may have diagnoses such as Attention Deficit Hyperactivity Disorder (ADHD) or Attachment Disorder or may have no formal diagnosis at all.

But what has that got to do with speech and language?

🏁 STARTING POINTS

Have you had experience of working with children and young people (CYP) with SEMH that you suspected had SLCN? How did you feel about this? What kinds of strategies did you implement at the time?

What are the key issues that you think these learners face in the school setting? What are the biggest risks?

What do you think makes the biggest difference for these CYP?

The relationship between SLCN and SEMH

It is well established in the research literature that there are high rates of SLCN amongst those with SEMH and vice versa (Levickis et al., 2018; Maggio et al., 2014;

Cohen et al., 2013). The interaction between these difficulties is complex (Conti-Ramsden et al., 2018) and for some it can be seen as a 'chicken and egg' situation – has the person developed SEMH over time because of unsupported SLCN? For example, has a learner's persistent unacknowledged difficulties understanding instructions led them to becoming anxious and withdrawn? Or is the reverse true – can SEMH lead to a CYP experiencing SLCN? For example, a learner with ADHD may find focusing on spoken instructions difficult, or a learner with Attachment Disorder may find initiating socially appropriate conversations challenging.

We know that positive communication skills are an important indicator of CYP wellbeing and a protective factor for resilience and mental health. Language is the medium in which we experience our thought processes, reasoning, decision-making and relationships with others, as well as how we make our needs, wants and feelings known. If a person has difficulty with this, it seems logical that it puts them at risk of negative physical and mental health experiences.

Unmet needs and negative life chances

SLCN in individuals with SEMH can often go unrecognised, undiagnosed and therefore unsupported (Hollo et al., 2014). Compounding this, behaviour can overshadow SLCN. For example, due to behaviour's more 'obvious' or 'risky' nature, teachers may be more focused on a learner disrupting a whole class's learning rather than an individual learner quietly struggling to understand their work.

Alternatively, even if staff do pick up on hidden SLCN, learners may not be seen as reaching thresholds for specialist referrals or staff perceive that specialist services won't take them on due to high waiting lists, so a referral is not made (McCool, 2023). Sometimes the specialist service requiring a referral can even be misidentified, for example learners get referred only to behaviour support rather than speech and language therapy (SaLT).

However, this persistent lack of support can unfortunately lead to various negative life effects:

- Vocabulary difficulties at age five are significantly associated with poor literacy, mental health and employment outcomes at age 34 (Law et al., 2009). See Chapters 7 and 8 for more information on this.
- 90% of care leavers had below average language abilities and over 60% met the criteria for a diagnosis of Developmental Language Disorder (DLD) (Clegg et al., 2021).
- Approximately 60% of young people involved with the criminal justice system have SLCN (Bryan et al., 2007).
- 88% of long-term unemployed young men have been found to have SLCN (Elliott, 2011).

It is clear that CYP with SEMH and SLCN do not 'grow out' of these issues. So how do they occur?

Trauma and SLCN

Negative life experiences are often labelled by professionals as adverse childhood experiences (ACEs). Exposure to ACEs, such as abuse and neglect, can result in changes to the brain, for example, chronic levels of exposure to stress hormones. Trauma can also create changes in the body and brain that can lead to SLCN:

So how do some of these issues start to manifest for learners? What is the starting point?

Attachment and SLCN

A key part of developing positive SEMH is the establishment of secure attachments, or a reliable bond between a person and their 'attachment figure' for safety, protection and comfort (Prior and Glaser, 2006). Positive, predictable and emotionally attuned relationships are needed for secure attachment, so energy can be spent exploring the world and growing (McGlinn in Jagoe and Walsh, 2020). When disruptive events or atypical attachments are formed, this can impact upon a CYP's communication.

Ainsworth (1978) found that there are four attachment styles: secure, insecure-anxious, insecure-avoidant and disorganised. CYPs with any of the three insecure attachment styles can engage in less reciprocal, or two-way, interactions. This gives the CYP fewer opportunities to participate in language-learning interactions with caregivers, with a knock-on negative impact on language development.

Securely attached CYP are more likely to have more effective communication skills, including emotional literacy and social interactions (Murray and Yingling, 2000). Table 11.2 explains how each attachment style can be linked to SLCN:

Table 11.1 The impact of trauma on a learner with corresponding SLCN

Impact of trauma on a child	Related SLCNs
Hyper-vigilance/hyper-arousal (on alert at all times)	Difficulty listening and focusing on what is being said Extra sensitive to negative comments or non-verbal communication (e.g. 'you looked at me funny')
Attachment difficulties (see following section)	Issues with maintaining socially appropriate conversations and relationships Passive and/or aggressive communication styles
Lack of exposure to typical communication styles	Less likely to express their thoughts, wants and needs Vulnerable to peer pressure and social exploitation

Table 11.2 Attachment styles and SLC profiles (based on Ainsworth's 1978 attachment styles)

Attachment style	Behaviour	SLC profile
Secure	Engages in learning Has appropriate peer relationships Emotionally regulated in line with their age	Able to follow instructions Can express wants, needs and feelings Engages in socialisation Sensitive to others' needs Seeks help when needed
Insecure-anxious	Fear of abandonment/rejection Seeks constant support Overfamiliar with strangers	Seeks repetitive interactions, e.g. reassurance Interaction is focused on seeking approval Misunderstanding of socially appropriate boundaries Susceptible to peer pressure and is overly compliant
Insecure-avoidant	Hyper-independent Doesn't ask for help Won't trust others Not close with others Won't share information	Difficulty with emotional vocabulary beyond basic negative words, e.g. 'anger' Communication may come across as blunt Dominant in expressing what is acceptable Prefer to be alone
Disorganised	Mixture of anxious and avoidant behaviours Anger with no obvious reason Hypervigilant Inconsistent in interaction with staff (caring vs aggression)	Mixture of the above as well as: Difficulty understanding intentions and needs of others May want to form relationships but sabotages them Difficulties focusing Extra sensitivity to non-verbal cues, e.g. tone of voice

ⓘ CRITICAL QUESTIONS

How does the above information relate to the CYP you work with?

What kinds of attachment styles do your learners with SEMH present with?

How have you seen trauma manifest in the communication skills of SEMH learners?

Identification is key

We have previously established that SLCN is prevalent, but often undetected in learners with SEMH and therefore professionals need to know how to identify it. The first step is making sure school staff are trained in this issue, from the senior leadership team to administration staff. Training can be completed in conjunction with local SaLT teams or via online resources (see end of chapter for suggestions).

Being able to recognise a potential SLCN is only the first step. Staff then need access to the tools to confirm their suspicions. SLCN screening tools are an important tool for non-SaLTs to do this. These include:

- Wellcomm
- Language Link
- Nuffield Early Language Intervention (NELI)
- Talk Boost
- The Communication Trust's Progression Tools.

Local initiatives may also be available and can be found, for example, on Local Offer and NHS SaLT websites.

Reframing SEMH as SLCN

Once a learner with SEMH's SLCN has been identified, professionals can plan how to support them. This sometimes involves reframing what was thought of as purely SEMH to include SLCN in the child's story. We'll now discuss some examples.

Pierre, primary, alternative provision (AP)

Consider a primary-aged mainstream pupil, Pierre. He presents in school as:

- struggling to hold a two-way conversation;
- whispering to himself repetitively;
- demonstrating excessive motor behaviours, e.g. waving his hands and running around;
- ceasing to verbally communicate whenever anyone approaches him and sits or stands as though frozen.

Pierre would run around school, disrupting other's learning along the way. Initially, staff perceived Pierre's difficulties as primarily SEMH. Early indicators suggested he required the input of a psychologist to unpick the emotional needs being displayed, with staff concerned it was childhood psychosis.

However, Pierre was able to focus on tasks he enjoyed, such as computer games. His teachers described him as being a 'computer whizz' when emotionally regulated and he

Table 11.3 An explanation of how behaviours thought to be psychosis were reframed as autism

Perceived as psychosis	Reframed as autism
Talking and laughing to himself	• Rehearsing sentences and repeating what has been said to him (echolalia) • Talking externally about things that made him laugh or that he found funny
Excessive motor behaviours, e.g. unable to remain in seat, waving his hands in front of screens, running and jumping around school	• Waving his hands was a form of stimming – often displayed when he was excited or happy • Pierre needed sensory breaks between tasks/activities within the classroom due to sensory and expectation overload • He required staff to support and facilitate his movement breaks to allow him time to better regulate himself, so that he would be able to move on to the next learning task in the classroom/expectation of him
Unable to follow societal norms when someone was talking/engaging with him	• No awareness of neurotypical social expectations and boundaries • He required explicit teaching of what are conventionally socially appropriate behaviours when with others, e.g. he would regularly look over a teacher's shoulder when they were typing

was able to use an aided language display to communicate during these times too. Pierre demonstrated that when given the right communication tools, he was able to engage with others.

Pierre, who was bilingual, displayed similar behaviours at home. Family perceived him as disruptive and unable to keep himself safe. It wasn't until Pierre was moved from his mainstream school to a pupil referral unit (PRU) that a referral was made to SaLT.

The results of a SaLT assessment allowed school staff to understand his communication profile and for a multi-agency differential diagnosis. Instead of continuing to pursue the diagnosis of childhood psychosis, an autism assessment was initiated instead. Professionals were able to reframe some of the behaviours listed above as neurodivergent rather than psychotic. Table 11.3 discusses this in more detail.

 CASE STUDY 1
Hayley, adolescent, alternative provision

Hayley was referred by her mainstream secondary school to an alternative provision (AP) in Year 11 due to issues managing her anxiety, including self-harm. Hayley had missed a significant amount of education because of this.

As she joined the AP, Hayley was situationally mute. This meant she was unable to speak at school and at home was verbally communicating with only select family members. She engaged in self-harming behaviours, as well as disordered eating and it also became apparent that Hayley had an extensive range of sensory needs.

Whilst in school, Hayley would rely on either head shakes or nods to communicate with a limited number of staff. With staff she didn't know, she would keep her head down, hair over her face and would not acknowledge them. Within class, she was bright and her written work demonstrated her ability to be articulate. Staff could have perceived Hayley's behaviour in school as non-compliance or that she was deliberately not engaging in school life.

However, after a referral to SaLT, Hayley was formally given a diagnosis of situational mutism and, later, a multi-agency diagnosis of autism, for her ongoing social communication needs and sensory profile.

Over time, she began to build trusted relationships with staff she saw regularly and was able to use a whispering voice to engage in two-way conversations. Taking the time to get to know Hayley, as well as creating ways for her to participate in lessons that weren't verbal, was paramount to building trusted relationships. She relied on these staff to support her when she experienced change. She received weekly mentoring and communication support to better explore her needs and for staff to gain clarity of what worked well for her specific needs.

Table 11.4 How behaviours thought to be anxiety were reframed as autism

Perceived as anxiety	*Reframed as autistic spectrum condition*
Would not contribute verbally to lessons or group work	• Hayley experienced difficulties knowing what to say and when Staff who had a trusted relationship with Hayley needed to recognise when her eye contact decreased because this indicated she needed a sensory break
Refusal to eat in front of others	• Hayley had sensory issues and struggled to eat in front of and amongst peers whilst they ate • She struggled with noises such as others chewing, yawning or coughing
Self-harm tendencies	• When Hayley experienced happiness or joy, she felt the need to harm – almost as if she felt guilty for experiencing those emotions • Staff provided a consistent emotion coaching approach to support her in school

CASE STUDY 2
TRAVIS, Year 7 pupil

An AP offered a place to a Year 7 pupil, Travis, who was due to be permanently excluded from his mainstream school for breaking the arm of a peer by dropping a heavy object down a flight of stairs. Travis claimed that he hadn't done anything wrong and appeared to find the event funny. He had a history of walking out of lessons, being rude to staff and demonstrated no awareness of danger for either himself or peers. At home, Travis displayed similar behaviours and his parents struggled to manage them.

Yet, it quickly became apparent that Travis struggled to access the language around him. He relied on phrases such as, 'What did you say?' and 'Why's he/she saying that to me?' when people spoke to him. When asked to explain what happened, he often explained things in a muddled-up order and needed additional adult support to help him order his school day. When he became overwhelmed, he would walk off or demonstrate 'anti-social' behaviours, such as swearing and shouting.

Travis was referred to the AP's SaLT for investigation. Assessments revealed that he struggled with both receptive and expressive language, he needed visuals to support his understanding of language and tasks to be broken down into manageable chunks with a 'task and finish' approach, giving him regular brain breaks during lessons to support his engagement.

Travis received a diagnosis of Developmental Language Disorder (DLD). Both home and school felt that this diagnosis supported Travis' needs. He needed additional support through an education, health and care plan, and he later gained a place in a specialist setting that could meet his needs.

Table 11.5: How behavioural difficulties were reframed as DLD

Perceived as behavioural issues	Reframed as DLD
Hurting/injuring peers	• Travis did not understand consequential behaviours for himself or others, i.e. 'if I throw this item, it could hurt another person'. He needed to be taught explicitly about how his actions could impact others.
Laughing or dismissing adults when being spoken to	• Poor receptive and expressive language skills meant that Travis was unable to access and comprehend what was being said to him. Without language being adapted to an accessible level with visual support, his go-to response to deflect attention away from him was to either laugh or walk away.

Table 11.5 (Continued)

Perceived as behavioural Issues	Reframed as DLD
Absconding from lessons/school buildings when dysregulated	• When Travis became overwhelmed with the language around him, it was easier for him to disengage and leave the classroom than remain in it. This was especially the case when he perceived staff as not understand his needs – he would say, 'he/she isn't helping me!' • Travis needed visual cues in his lessons to help support his understanding. He also benefited from staff explaining words to him in a 1:1 context – however, he was also sensitive to how his peers viewed his 1:1 support. The staff he formed trusted relationships with knew to provide him with subtle support without him feeling embarrassed for needing extra help.

⑦ Critical questions

a) Do any of these case studies resonate with you and the CYP you've worked with?

b) What strategies were put in place for those learners? How effective were they?

c) Where do you think the gaps were for these students and how did this impact on the behaviours you were seeing if they became dysregulated and/or overstimulated?

STRATEGIES FOR ADAPTIVE PLANNING

The aim for those with SEMH and SLCN is to make language clear and not open to misinterpretation, to lessen anxiety, manage expectations and increase independence.

1. **Complete a 'communication-friendly' environment audit.** Tools such as the Communication Supporting Classroom Observation Tool (Dockrell et al., 2012) can be used to assess the effectiveness of the language-learning environment, opportunities and interactions within your setting. You can then set goals on areas you want to improve as the term progresses.

2. **Visual cues** are a useful strategy to support all learners and are a quick, time-effective way to support focus and understanding. Table 11.6 details ways of implementing this:

3. **Language adaptation** can support a CYP's engagement in conversation and learning. Staff should be mindful of the length and complexity of the instructions and information they are providing verbally. Simplify wording where possible, and when using complex curriculum vocabulary use visual

Table 11.6 Key visuals and their purpose

Resource	Purpose
Visual timetables	To allow pupils to know what is happening, orient themself in time and predict what is next.
Task boards	To show what is expected in a task or lesson, including equipment required, and clearly predict the finish point.
Aided language display or communication book	To clearly show vocabulary that can be used, allow for creation of longer sentences and model how language can be used.
Word webs or mind maps	To support understanding and retention of new vocabulary and concepts (see Chapter 7 for more information on this)

supports for dual coding as outlined above. Chunk sentences into key parts and again support them with a visual, e.g. writing it on the board at the same time. See Chapter 13 for a full list of adaptation strategies to support this cohort. These adaptations prevent learners with SEMH and SLCN becoming overwhelmed, overstimulated and disengaged. Successful completion of smaller, accessible tasks will foster motivation and a willingness to achieve further.

4. **Be inclusive in your acceptance of different social skills**. For example, eye contact should not be a prerequisite for learning or conversations. The demand to give eye contact can place unnecessary and excessive emotional strain on a learner. Some learners will focus so much on providing eye contact that they are then unable to follow what is being discussed in the lesson and unable to start their work. For other learners, the need to provide eye contact will cause them to experience physical and emotional discomfort. Staff need to acknowledge that just because a CYP is engaging differently, does not mean they aren't paying attention or not wanting to be in their classroom. For teachers to get the best from their pupils, learners need to feel safe and secure in their learning environment.

5. When difficult social situations occur, explore them visually, e.g. using **Comic Strip Conversations** (Gray, 1994). These allow CYP to slowly describe and reflect on what happened and allows them and staff to understand.

It is important that staff also identify the CYP who will require additional interventions beyond what is available universally for all learners in order for them to engage and achieve. SaLT teams will be able to provide more information about recommended interventions. Programmes such as Talkabout (Kelly, 2018) have shown good progress rates amongst pupils.

📝 CHAPTER SUMMARY

This chapter has outlined the link between SLCN and SEMH for CYP. Whilst it is little known amongst the general public, pupils with SEMH often have undiagnosed SLCN and vice versa.

It is crucial that school staff are well equipped with the knowledge to recognise this in their learners, and have access to screening tools to identify the needs and practical strategies to support these often-vulnerable CYP.

This chapter isn't able to cover all of the knowledge, tools and strategies available to school staff, so, therefore, please see below links to further information on this topic.

📖 Further Reading

Branagan, A, Parsons, S, and Cross, M (2020). *Language for Behaviour and Emotions: A Practical Guide to Working with Pupil and Young People* (1st edition). Routledge. https://doi.org/10.4324/9780429318320

This text covers more detailed information on SLCN and SEMH and includes a screening tool and intervention programme to be used with pupils.

McLachlan, H and Elks, L (2023) *Elklan Language Builders for Social, Emotional and Mental Health*, Elklan, SALT Training Consultants.

Read this text to learn practical strategies to support pupils with SEMH and SLCN in the school environment.

RCSLT (2023) *Mind Your Words*. Available: www.rcslt.org/learning/mind-your-words/ [Accessed: 09.11.2024].

This is free online learning with 15 modules on supporting pupils with SEMH and SLCN to reach their full potential.

📚 References

Ainsworth, M D S (1978) The Bowlby-Ainsworth attachment theory. *The Behavioral and Brain Sciences*, 1(3): 436–438. https://doi.org/10.1017/S0140525X00075828

Bryan, K, Freer, J, and Furlong, C (2007) Language and communication difficulties in juvenile offenders. *International Journal of Language & Communication Disorders*, 42(5): 505–520. https://doi.org/10.1080/13682820601053977

Clegg, J, Crawford, E, Spencer, S, and Matthews, D (2021). Developmental language disorder (DLD) in young people leaving care in England: A study profiling the language, literacy and communication abilities of young people transitioning from care to independence. *International Journal of Environmental Research and Public Health*, 18(8): 4107. https://doi.org/10.3390/ijerph18084107

Cohen, N J, Farnia, F, and Im-Bolter, N (2013) Higher order language competence and adolescent mental health. *Journal of Pupil Psychology and Psychiatry*. 54(7): 733–744.

Conti-Ramsden, G, Durkin, K, Toseeb, U, Botting, N, and Pickles, A (2018) Education and employment outcomes of young adults with a history of developmental language disorder. *International Journal of Language & Communication Disorders*, 53(2): 237–255. https://doi.org/10.1111/1460-6984.12338

Department for Education (2024) *Special educational needs in England*. Available here: www.explore-education-statistics.service.gov.uk/find-statistics.special-educational-needs-in-england [Accessed: 09.11.2024].

Department for Education and Department of Health (2015) *Special educational needs and disability code of practice: 0 to 25 years*. Available at: www.gov.uk/government/publications/send-code-of-practice-0-to-25 [Accessed: 09.11.2024].

Dockrell, J, Bakopoulou, I, Law, J, Spencer, S, and Lindsay, G (2012) Communication Supporting Classroom Observation Tool, The Communication Trust. Available at: https://www.hertsgovernors.org/wp-content/uploads/2014/10/Communication-Supporting-Classroom-Observation-Tool.pdf [Accessed: 25.01.25].

Elliott, N L (2011) *An Investigation Into the Communication Skills of Unemployed Young Men*. ProQuest Dissertations & Theses.

Gray, C (1994) *Comic Strip Conversations*. Arlington, TX: New Horizons, Inc.

Hollo, A, Wehby, J H, and Oliver, R M (2014) Unidentified Language Deficits in Pupil with Emotional and Behavioral Disorders: A MetaAnalysis. *Exceptional Pupil*; 80(2): 169–186.

Kelly, A (2018) *Talkabout: A Social Communication Skills Package*. Taylor & Francis Group https://doi.org/10.4324/9781315173849

Law, J, Rush, R, Schoon, I, and Parsons, S (2009) Modeling developmental language difficulties from school entry into adulthood: Literacy, mental health, and employment outcomes. *Journal of Speech, Language, and Hearing Research*, 52(6): 1401–1416. https://doi.org/10.1044/1092-4388(2009/08-0142)

Levickis, P, Sciberras, E, McKean, C, Conway, L, Peziic, A, Mensah, F K, Bavin, E L, Bretherton, L, Eadie, P, Prior, M, and Reilly, S (2018) Language and social-emotional and behavioural wellbeing from 4 to 7 years: A community-based study. *European Pupil Adolescent Psychiatry*. 27: 849–859. https://doi.org/10.1007/s00787-017-1079-7

Maggio, V, Grañana, N E, Richaudeau, A, Torres, S, Giannotti, A, and Suburo, A M (2014) Behavior problems in pupil with specific language impairment. *Journal of Pupil Neurology*, 29(2): 194–202. https://doi.org/10.1177/0883073813509886

McCool, S (2023) *Working with Pupil and Adolescent Mental Health: The Central Role of Language and Communication* (1st ed., Vol. 1). Routledge. https://doi.org/10.4324/9781003258476

McGlinn, S (2020) Communication and infant mental health. In Jagoe, C, and Walsh, I P (Eds.) (2020) *Communication and mental health disorders: Developing theory, growing practice*. J&R Press Ltd.

Murray, A D and Yingling, J L (2000) Competence in language at 24 months: Relations with attachment security and home stimulation. *The Journal of Genetic Psychology: Research and Theory on Human Development*, 161(2): 133–140. https://doi.org/10.1080/00221320009596700

Prior, V, and Glaser, D (2006) *Understanding Attachment and Attachment Disorders: Theory, Evidence and Practice*. Jessica Kingsley Publishers.

12 Speech, language and communication needs in the school exclusion process

Claire Westwood and Helen Knowler

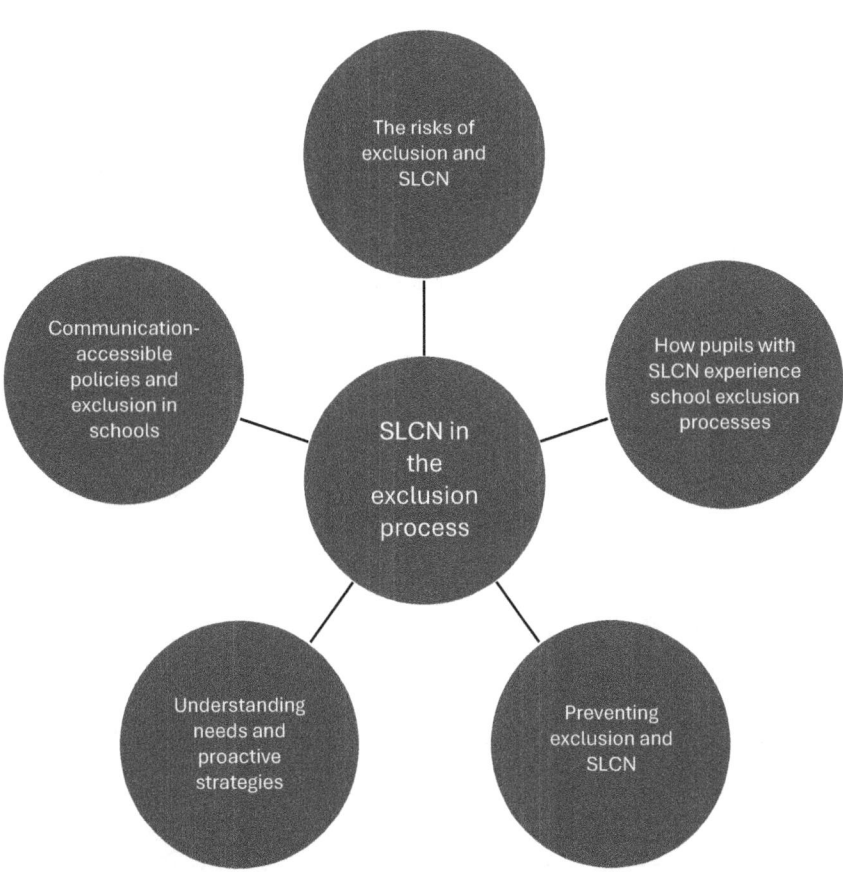

DOI: 10.4324/9781041054986-15

CHAPTER OBJECTIVES

This chapter explores the relationship between speech, language and communication needs (SLCN) and school exclusion. It will:

- introduce you to the relationship between SLCN and school exclusion practices and processes;
- enable you to reflect on your experience of supporting pupils with SLCN and understanding their risk of school exclusion;
- use critical questions to support you to identify the key challenges and responses when working to prevent the exclusion of pupils with SLCN;
- self-check and offer resources that can support your development and practice in this area.

Introduction

It may not be immediately clear why SLCN is related to school exclusion. Children who get excluded can talk and get themselves into trouble, right?

Whilst it is well established in research that the main cause of school exclusion is persistent disruptive behaviour (Department for Education, 2023/2024), there is a strong link between behavioural difficulties and undiagnosed SLCN (Anderson, Hawes and Snow, 2016). Studies show that 50–100% of children excluded, or at risk of exclusion, experience difficulties with understanding, processing and using spoken language (Clegg et al., 2009, Ripley and Yuill, 2005).

This chapter will outline how SLCN can trigger and/or impact upon a child's experiences of school exclusion processes, such as:

- managed moves;
- entry to a pupil referral unit (PRU);
- or transfer to alternative provision (AP).

We also want to highlight the increased risk of exposure to criminality outside school when children with SLCN experience exclusionary processes in schools (Done & Knowler, 2023).

STARTING POINTS

- Have you had experience of working with excluded pupils who had SLCN? If so, how did you feel about this? Do you think the pupil understood their exclusion and its processes?

- Have you seen good examples of prevention work for pupils at risk of exclusion? What factors seem to make the biggest difference?
- Do you know of initiatives in your setting that support dialogue about how to support excluded pupils with SLCN?

Overview of school exclusion and the link to SLCN

School exclusion is a persistent feature of the school disciplinary landscape, and it is common for schools in England to see exclusion as a necessary process for maintaining discipline in the wider school setting. The use of exclusion in school is controversial (Thompson, 2023) with differing views about the ways that exclusion should be used. Daniels et al. (2023) argue that school exclusion should be understood holistically as something that impacts on and is impacted by education, health and welfare. Others relate exclusion simply as an outcome of behaviour infringement and therefore a logical consequence of a failure to adjust to expectations of behaviour and learning. However exclusion is conceptualised, there is no doubt that its impacts can be devasting for pupils, their families and education professionals involved in exclusions (Zhang et al., 2024).

Exclusion in schools can come in many shapes and guises. In English schools, exclusion can be fixed term (a suspension) or permanent (removal from school setting). An exclusion should only be given for disciplinary reasons but as outlined below this is very vague and recent evidence suggests that some pupils seem more at risk of exclusion than others, such as those with special educational needs and disabilities (SEND) and those from specific ethnic groups (for example, see Demie, 2019). Only a headteacher can exclude a pupil on disciplinary grounds. According to the DfE (2024) guidance, a headteacher should consider the views of pupils when deciding whether they exclude and this should be done considering their age and understanding.

As above, a significant proportion of excluded children and young people (CYP) have difficulties understanding, processing and using spoken language. For example, RCSLT (2017) found that **90%** of the entrants to a pupil referral unit in the London Borough of Newham presented with moderate-significant SLCN upon assessment and only a small number of these had previously had their SLCN identified. This can be important when considering heavily verbally mediated exclusion processes, e.g. meetings discussing behaviour incidents and agreeing to conditions of a managed move.

Before we reach this point, what we often see as speech and language therapists (SaLTs) is that some children with social emotional mental health needs (SEMH) and (often undiagnosed) SLCN can cope within a supportive primary school setting. The fact they only must manage one classroom environment and one teacher, who often knows them really well, means that there are fewer obstacles to overcome.

This relates to the demands and capacities model (Starkweather et al., 1990), i.e. the internal goings-on for a person (their capacities) being unbalanced by the external pressure put onto them (the demands). The demands of the secondary school environment start to outweigh a child with SLCN and SEMH's capacity to process information, regulate their emotions and express themselves. This can then lead to behaviours that challenge and trigger the slide down the school-to-prison pipeline, aka the pushing of vulnerable children out of education and into the criminal justice system, starting with school exclusion.

What is also seen is the mislabelling of CYP with SLCN and SEMH as 'naughty', 'lazy' or 'un-cooperative', as outlined in Chapter 11. This is compounded by the fact that SLCN is an invisible disability, i.e. difficult to spot unless you know what you are looking for (Griffiths et al., 2024). In schools, behaviour policies are often verbally mediated and orthographically circulated, i.e. students are told about them and they are stuck on the wall in a way those with SLCN find difficult to understand and retain. McGregor (2020) notes how isolating it can feel for pupils who do not understand the rules and regulations and this leads to a lack of support or resources for their inclusion.

ⓘ CRITICAL QUESTIONS

- How does a member of staff explain to a child how they need to change their behaviour?
- How does a member of the senior leadership team tell the child they're being excluded?
- How do schools inform a child of the conditions of a managed move?

SPOTLIGHT ON NEW DEBATES: INFORMAL AND UNLAWFUL EXCLUSION

The formal process of exclusion in schools is clearly outlined in the Department for Education's Behaviour and Attendance policies (DfE, 2024). However, since 2017 there have been a range of concerns about the use of exclusion to manipulate pupil populations and to create the impression that a school is 'high performing' in league tables and therefore more likely to get a more favourable Ofsted rating. Researchers have demonstrated that there are a range of informal, and sometimes unlawful, exclusionary practices whereby pupils are informally excluded (Done et al., 2021) on a fixed-term basis or where pupils move into another provision without an adequate assessment of whether this meets their needs. This 'dark side' of inclusion (Soan, 2006) raises serious questions about the ability of schools to fully support pupils with SEND, and more specifically SLCN, and whilst assumed that this is done inadvertently or with good intentions, not all researchers think this is the case (Done et al., 2021) when the phenomenon can be seen in other countries across the globe.

The key issue with informal (and potentially unlawful) exclusionary practices is that they often look like good strategies for coping with challenging behaviour. Examples of informal practices can be as straightforward as sending home a pupil at lunchtime to 'cool off', to the use of an informal part-time timetable or extensive use of 'inclusion' rooms. The strategies can be used in the best interests of the setting, rather than the best interests of the pupils. These strategies become unlawful if they are not recorded by the school or are done on an informal basis without recourse to a formal process. An example of unlawful practice is 'off rolling', which is the exclusion of a pupil based on their academic performance. However, there has been evidence of schools 'gaming' the system so that the pupils with the lowest academic performances are moved out and therefore so that they are not included in performance data. It is easy to imagine that pupils with SLCN (that is often unidentified), and those who are not performing well in formal assessments, could be targeted in this way. The pandemic exacerbated the issue of informal and unlawful exclusion as schools adjusted to provision on site and online.

 CRITICAL REFLECTION

The Education Policy Institute (2019) stated that pupils more likely to experience an unexplained exit from school include:

over 1 in 3 (36.2%) of all pupils who had also experienced a permanent exclusion;

around 1 in 3 (29.8%) of all looked after pupils (those in social care);

over 1 in 4 (27.0%) of all pupils with identified mental health needs (SEMH);

around 1 in 6 (15.6%) of all poorer pupils (those who have ever been on free school meals);

around 1 in 6 (15.7%) of all pupils with identified SEND;

around 1 in 7 (13.9%) of all pupils from Black ethnic backgrounds.

- How can educators advocate for pupils in these groups and be vigilant to the exclusionary experiences they might have in schools?

Everything happens verbally

So many parts to the legal exclusions process require a high level of verbal competence for the pupils and families involved and it can be easy to miss signs that SLCN may be a contributory factor to the escalation of an incident. Table 12.1 illustrates how this may occur:

172 • Developing Speech, Language and Communication Skills in Education

Table 12.1 The link between legal actions that may result in exclusion and hidden SLCN

Action that schools may lawfully exclude a child for	How it might be SLCN
Repeated failure to follow academic instruction	Difficulty with receptive language or processing spoken information Doesn't realise they've misunderstood No strategy to ask for help in a productive way Misunderstanding and difficulty using emotional vocabulary
Failure to complete a behavioural sanction, e.g. detention	Can't tell the time Unable to organise themselves independently, e.g. keep track of commitments Lack of consequential thinking abilities
Repeated and persistent breaches of the school's behavioural policy	Doesn't understand the vocabulary or complex sentence structures used in the behaviour policy Can't read the behaviour policy Doesn't understand the consequences of not following the rules Consequential thinking issues related to sanctions or negative outcomes No strategies to ask for help
Inappropriate responses to direction or modification from teachers or peers	Social communication differences Hasn't understood the instruction Wasn't able to maintain attention to the direction

CASE STUDY

Tyler is in Year 10 and just got into a fight at school as another child teased him for taking something literally. Tyler quickly got angry and hit the child. The assistant head saw this happen and sent Tyler home. Tyler's mother asks him what happened and he says he can't remember because he was so upset. The next week, the school invite Tyler and his Mum into school to discuss a managed move as this is the third fight Tyler has been in this term. Tyler can't keep up with what the adults are talking about so becomes silent. When asked what he thinks, he has no idea how to explain his point of view so shrugs his shoulders. Tyler's difficulties understanding, processing and using spoken language mean he hasn't been able to participate in his managed move process. Instead, adults have had to make decisions for him and he doesn't understand the conditions involved. This places the managed move at risk of breakdown.

We know that verbally based interventions are difficult to access for young people who have SLCN (Sirianni, 2004). Under the Equality Act (2010) schools have a duty to make reasonable adjustments, including to exclusion processes.

For Tyler this could have looked like:

- The use of a Comic Strip Conversation (Gray, 1994) after he has calmed down from the behavioural incident to explore what happened and how amends could be made.
- A communication-accessible behaviour policy, perhaps adhering to Easy Read principles, that Tyler is actually able to understand and process.
- The use of Talking Mats before the meeting to enable his voice to be heard regarding the options available to him. Find out more about Talking Mats at talkingmats.com.
- Simplified language, symbol-supported conversation and a visual agenda during the meeting to ensure Tyler's full participation, understanding and expression in what was going on.

This chapter will now go on to discuss more practical ways school staff can support children with SLCN at risk of exclusion.

STRATEGIES FOR SUPPORT

There are many supportive strategies that school staff can implement to support CYP with SEMH at risk of, or going through, school exclusion. First, it is important to consider SLCN as a contributory factor in all school exclusions. The below checklist can be used as an informal guide to this (Table 12.2):

Table 12.2 Reflective checklist to consult before excluding

Y/N	Factor to consider
	Has the child been screened for SLCN? If SLCN has been picked up at screen, have the relevant SaLT services been approached to assess and has time been given for post-screening strategies to be implemented?
	Are you confident that the child has been able to access the language within the school's behaviour policies and processes? Can this child's behaviour be explained by an inability to understand/process an instruction? Or by social interaction challenges? Does the child understand why they have been excluded? Can they explain this back to you? Does the child understand the conditions of their exclusion or managed move? Can they explain this back to you?
	Has this child had communication access provided to put forward their perspective and understand other's perspectives as part of the exclusion process?

(Continued)

Table 12.2 *(Continued)*

Y/N	Factor to consider
	If on a managed move, has SLCN been integrated into the planning process?
	Do you have alternative methods to enable a pupil to communicate their views and experiences, such as visuals of processes and choices on offer?

Communication-accessible documentation

Communication-accessible behaviour policies and contracts are another key part of ensuring CYP with SLCN are not disproportionately excluded. This may look like using simplified or Easy Read language, or even symbol-supported text. More information on Easy Read can be found on mencap.co.uk.

An example of a behaviour contract as used in Youth Justice can be seen in Figure 12.1.

Additional documentation that can be made in this format include:

– Preparation and minutes from exclusion or transition meetings
– Letters outlining details of exclusions
– Managed move contracts

Training

It is crucial that all the professionals around a child have the knowledge to identify and put in basic supports for SLCN. Free online training exists in this area, such as the RCSLT's Mind Your Words or The Box training which can be found on www.rcslt.org.

Local speech and language therapy teams can also offer training in understanding the link between SLCN and behaviour and providing more strategies and resources to support this. For example, the workbook 'Language of Behaviour and Emotions' (Branagan et al., 2021) or advocating the use of apps such as 'Mind of my Own' which help a CYP's voice be heard in meetings.

De-escalation strategies

The following key strategies can support CYP with SLCN to be able to participate in behaviour and exclusions processes.

Attention/Listening

1. Say the CYP's name to cue them into what you're saying, before giving them an instruction.

Speech, language and communication needs • **175**

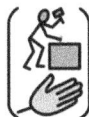

Reparation hours:

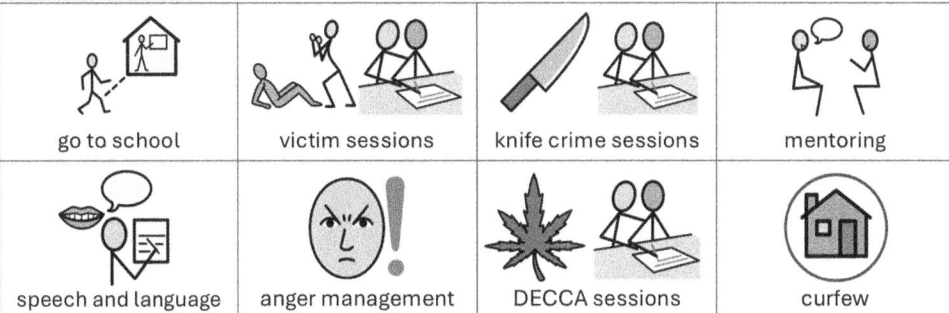

I also need to:

go to school	victim sessions	knife crime sessions	mentoring
speech and language	anger management	DECCA sessions	curfew

I will finish this by:

Signed:

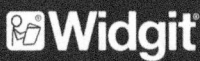 This resource was created using Widgit Symbols. Widgit Symbols ©Widgit Software Ltd. 2002-2025.   Create your own visit **widgit.com**

Figure 12.1 *A communication-accessible contract made in Sandwell Youth Justice service by author Claire Westwood (Permission to reproduce the Widgit Symbols © Widgit Software Ltd. 2002–2025 granted by Anna Cawrey, partnerships manager, Widgit, March 2025)*

2. Set clear expectations about what you need from them at the start of sessions or meetings. Provide these visually in the form of a task plan or a list; e.g. 'This meeting will last 20 minutes, and we will talk about X, Y and Z'. Get the CYP to tick them off they are completed.

3. Set breaks in sessions and meetings and support them to identify what they need to do to re-regulate, e.g. go for a walk.

4. Accept different and inclusive ways of listening – some neurodivergent children will still be listening even though they are not making eye contact, other children may need to keep moving or fidgeting but are still listening.

Behaviour/Emotional regulation

1. Be consistent, kind, honest and clear in how you communicate with students.

2. Give CYP regular and specific feedback on what they have done right, not just what you need them to change.

3. Keep CYP informed of what is happening and why.

4. When a CYP is upset or angry, allow them time to calm down before you expect them to reflect on their actions or problem solve. As outlined in Chapter 4, often in the heat of the moment CYP can't reflect 'on the spot' so it is beneficial to let them re-regulate first.

5. When doing the reflective work afterwards, do this in a visual format such as a Comic Strip Conversation (Gray, 1994) to allow the CYP to understand everyone's point of view and express their perspective.

6. CYP often go through times when communicating is easier/harder than others which may be due to a variety of factors. Look out for signs that CYP are finding things difficult and alter your communication accordingly. These signs might be verbal (e.g. swearing or giving one-word answers) or non-verbal (e.g. closed body language or becoming restless) and the responsibility is with adults to identify these rather than expecting the child to do this.

7. Give CYP extra time to think about what has been said. If asking them to make a decision, provide all the options in a visual format then give them time to process and come back to you with their decision.

Conversations and supporting understanding

1. Keep your sentences short, simple and to the point– no jargon!

2. Allow CYP with SLCN extra thinking time when you have asked them a question. Count to ten in your head before repeating yourself. Silence is ok!

3. No abstract or non-literal language, e.g. sayings, sarcasm and metaphors.

4. Be factual and explicit – do not expect CYP with SLCN to 'read between the lines' or infer a message as this is something they can find challenging.

5. Don't assume a CYP has interpreted a social situation correctly, e.g. they may have taken sarcasm literally. Instead, explain things explicitly to them without judgement. For example, 'you did x, that made x sad' or 'I can see you're upset from your facial expression'.

6. Check a CYP's understanding of what you tell them by getting them to repeat back what you have said. DO NOT ask, 'do you understand?'

7. If a CYP's response to a question seems unusual or out of context, it may that they have interpreted it literally. It would help to pause, reword the question more simply and then try again. Bear in mind that the CYP could be embarrassed by this misunderstanding so try to be relaxed and respectful when re-asking the question.

8. During key conversations, use meaningful and age-appropriate visuals to support what is being said. For example, if explaining a situation, the adult can draw a simple line drawing whilst talking. Stick figures work, it doesn't have to be a masterpiece!

There are key times in a pupil's school career that the above strategies can be implemented to prevent exclusions. The figure below shows five of these key times where considering SLCN could block the school-to-prison pipeline (Figure 12.2).

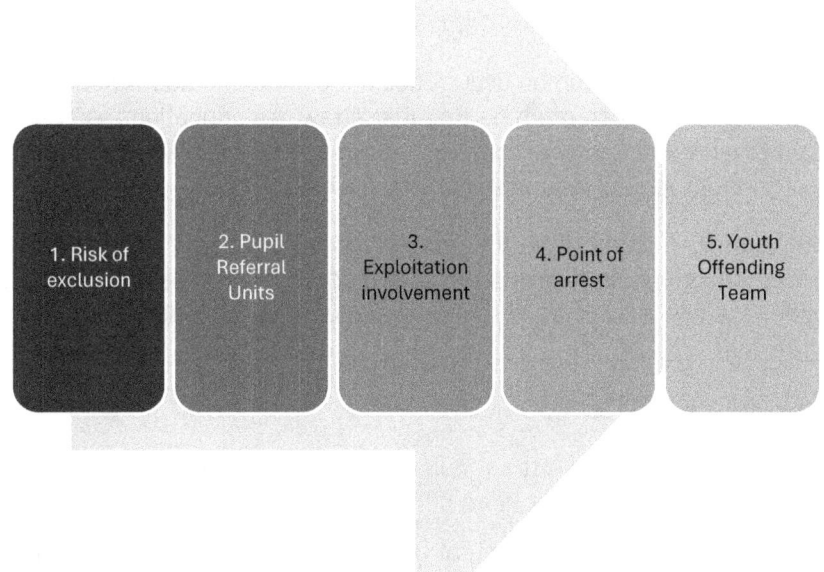

Figure 12.2 *Five stages at which it is important to consider SLCN as a contributory factor to block the school-to-prison pipeline (Westwood, 2021)*

CASE STUDIES

Let's now consider some real-life examples.

Cameron

Cameron is 13 years old and is in Year 8 at St Mary's Secondary School. Cameron was late to learn to talk as a toddler but caught up by the time he was in Year 2. He loves PE at school and is a keen footballer at the weekends.

Since starting secondary school, Cameron has made a reputation for himself as hard-to-teach. Teachers dread when they find out he is in their lesson as he often gets out of his seat and disrupts other students. He is always off-task and doesn't respond well to being told off.

The final straw is when Cameron swears at his English teacher and walks out when she asks him to read aloud in class. Cameron receives yet another suspension and teachers are deciding if this will be a permanent exclusion.

SaLT assessment shows that he has significant difficulties understanding multi-step instructions and doesn't have any productive strategies to ask for help. Assessment shows his vocabulary is significantly lower than expected for his age too.

In this example we can see the issue with cumulative behaviour issues resulting in Cameron's potential exclusion. Whilst no issue in isolation warrants permanent exclusion, the combination of in-class behaviour and the breakdown of relationships means that the school's capacity to support Cameron is diminished.

For example, swearing is a common occurrence in schools and so they show up in behaviour sanctions regularly. It can often be the 'last straw' for education professionals when they have observed persistently disruptive behaviour. However, we also know that Cameron lacks other appropriate vocabulary to ask for help.

A useful first step is to ensure that there is an agreement about a safe exit strategy for Cameron to re-regulate before re-entering the classroom. For pupils with SLCN this is useful provided visually as well as verbally, and when it is practised and rehearsed.

> **? CRITICAL QUESTIONS**
>
> - Why is Cameron off-task on a regular basis? Is he having difficultly accessing the curriculum and does he need differentiated tasks to experience success?
> - How can staff be supported so that they do not dread teaching Cameron – how can relationships be repaired and rebuilt?
> - What strategies can be used to support Cameron to understand classroom agreements and what are alternative methods for applying sanctions if required?

Bilal

Bilal is seven years old and has been temporarily suspended from his primary school for the second time. Bilal is known as a very likeable and outgoing child who can sometimes become overstimulated and verbally aggressive to staff.

Upon his return to school, his teacher talks to him about how his behaviour must be now he's back. Bilal listens intently to the new rules and says he'll try his best. She asks him, 'Now, how are you going to make sure this doesn't happen again?' and Bilal replies, 'You're so nosy, can't you just leave me alone!!' and storms off.

His teacher sees this as a 'red flag' and asks for support from the school's SaLT. The SaLT explains Bilal's latest assessment results that show Bilal doesn't understand 'how?' and 'why?' questions. These require abstract problem-solving and Bilal's defence mechanism is to deflect away from his lack of understanding and to escape the conversation.

We can see here that Bilal clearly has difficulties understanding spoken language and that behavioural strategies in this classroom are being verbally mediated.

Instead, the teacher and SaLT could plan how to adapt classroom questioning into a level that Bilal can process and understand (see Chapter 7). Next time they could ask Bilal 'Tell me the classroom rules we've talked about, please' instead, with reference to a visual representation of these rules. Perhaps then Bilal will be able to repeat back the necessary information showing he understands.

📝 CHAPTER SUMMARY

In this chapter we have argued that SLCN can have a significant impact on pupils' experiences of school behaviour systems that lead to school exclusion. We have shown that SLCN can be a significant factor in the range of reasons why pupils are excluded – particularly when undiagnosed.

We have explored the ways that some CYP have barriers to understanding and engaging with school behaviour processes, and even more problematic engagements with exclusion systems. We have explained the idea of the school-to-prison pipeline and how the cumulative impacts of what seem like behaviour infractions can lead to the idea that a pupil must leave a school based on their behaviour.

However, we have shown that there are a range of frameworks, tools and practices that can support inclusive provision and support you to ask critical questions if you suspect that SLCN is behind perceived behaviour issues. This can also help you to advocate for pupils to prevent exclusion of any kind. We know that supported, well trained and confident professionals are a crucial part of creating inclusive settings where there is little or no need for exclusion to happen at all.

Further reading/resources

- Royal College of Speech and Language Therapists (RCSLT)'s factsheet 'SLCN in Alternative Provision' gives an overview of the difference supporting SLCN can make in AP settings and can be read for free on rcslt.org.
- RCSLT have also put together a dossier of evidence on SLCN and exclusions again on the above website titled 'Exclusions review'.
- To hear what young people think about this topic, read 'Youth Voice: SEND and School Exclusions' by the Children's Society available for free on localgov.co.uk.

References

Anderson, S A S, Hawes, D J, and Snow, P C (2016) Language impairments among youth offenders: A systematic review. *Children and Youth Services Review*, 65: 195–203.

Branagan, A, Cross, M, and Parsons, S. (2021) *Language for Behaviour and Emotions: A Practical Guide to Working with Children and Young People*. 1st edition. Oxford: Routledge.

Clegg, J, Stackhouse, J, Finch, K, Murphy, C, and Nicholls, S. (2009) Language abilities of secondary age pupils at risk of school exclusion: A preliminary report. *Child Language Teaching and Therapy*, 25(1): 123–139. https://doi.org/10.1177/0265659008098664

Daniels, H, Thompson, I, and Emery, H (2023) Difference and school exclusion in a time of COVID-19. *International Journal of Inclusive Education*, 1–17. https://doi.org/10.1080/13603116.2023.2274110

Demie, F (2019) The experience of Black Caribbean pupils in school exclusion in England. *Educational Review*, 73(1): 55–70. https://doi.org/10.1080/00131911.2019.1590316

Department for Education (2023/24). Suspensions and permanent exclusions in England. Available here: https://explore-education-statistics.service.gov.uk/find-statistics.suspensions-and-permanent-exclusions-in-england [Accessed 24 February 2025).

Department for Education (2024) School suspensions and permanent exclusions - GOV.UK (Accessed 24 February 2025).

Done, E J and Knowler, H (Eds.) (2023) *International Perspectives on Exclusionary Pressures in Education: How Inclusion Becomes Exclusion*. Springer Nature.

Done, E J, Knowler, H, Shield, W, and Baynton, H (2021) Rocks and hard places: exploring educational psychologists' perspectives on "off-rolling" or illegal exclusionary practices in mainstream secondary schools in England. *Educational Psychology Research and Practice*, 7(2): 1–12.

Educational Policy Unit (EPI). (2019) Unexplained pupil exits from schools https://epi.org.uk/publications-and-research/unexplained-pupil-exits-data-multi-academy-trust-local-authority/

Equality Act 2010, c. 15. Available at: https://www.legislation.gov.uk/ukpga/2010/15/section/20 [Accessed 28 August 2025].

Gray, C (1994) *Comic strip conversations: illustrated interactions that teach conversation skills to students with autism and related disorders*. Rev. and updated. Arlington, TX: Future Horizons.

Griffiths, S, Lucas, L, Gooch, D, and Norbury, C F (2024) Special educational needs provision and academic outcomes for children with teacher reported language difficulties at school entry. *JCPP Advances*, e12264. https://doi.org/10.1002/jcv2.12264

McGregor, K K (2020) How we fail children with developmental language disorder. *Language, Speech, and Hearing Services in Schools*, 51(4): 981–992.

RCSLT (Royal College of Speech and Language Therapists). (2017) Exclusions review: Call for evidence. Available here: https://www.rcslt.org/wp-content/uploads/media/Project/RCSLT/exclusions-review-rcslt-written-evidence.pdf (accessed 24 February 2025).

Ripley, K and Yuill, N (2005) Patterns of language impairment and behaviour in boys excluded from school. *British Journal of Educational Psychology*, 75(1): 37–50. https://doi.org/10.1348/000709905X27696

Sirianni, J P (2004) Psychological stress and language processing in school-aged children. *Journal of Speech-Language Pathology and Audiology*. 28(3): 112–121.

Soan, S (2006) Are the needs of children and young people with social, emotional and behavioural needs being served within a multi-agency framework? *Support for learning*, 21(4): 210–215.

Starkweather, C W, Gottwald, S R, and Halfond, M M (1990). Stuttering prevention: A clinical method. Englewood Cliffs, NJ: Prentice-Hall.

Thompson I (2023). School exclusion, inclusion, and diversity: implications for initial teacher education. In Craig, C J, Mena, J, and Kane, R (Eds.) *Studying Teaching and Teacher Education* (*Advances in Research on Teaching*, Vol. 44), Leeds: Emerald Publishing Limited, pp. 315–327. https://doi.org/10.1108/S1479-368720230000044030.

Westwood, C (2021) *Using Speech and Language Therapy to Block the School-to-prison Pipeline*. Presented at the RCSLT Conference. London: United Kingdom.

Zhang, K, Tawell, A, and Evans-Lacko, S (2024) Full article: The costs of school exclusion: a case study analysis of England, Wales and Scotland. *Oxford Review of Education*, 50(6): 777–797 (accessed 24 February 2025).

SECTION III IMPLEMENTATION AND MOVING FORWARD

13 Preparation for adulthood
Aaron Emmett

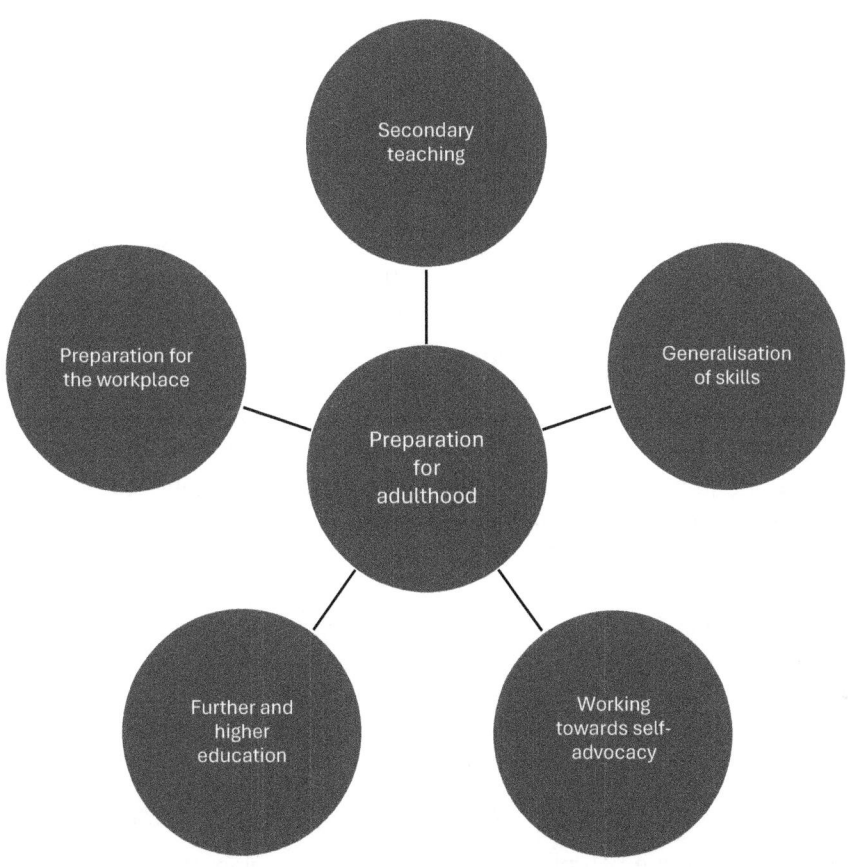

CHAPTER OBJECTIVES

This chapter looks to the future and explores how we can prepare children and young people with speech, language, and communication needs (SLCN) for adulthood. The chapter:

- explores how the education environment changes at secondary school and beyond for pupils with SLCN;
- considers how we can equip pupils with skills they can generalise to different areas of their life in and out of education, including skills for the workplace;
- suggests ways pupils can begin to understand their own needs and advocate for adjustments;
- proposes measures that further education and higher education institutions can use to meet the needs of learners with SLCN.

Introduction

As detailed in previous chapters (6, 7, 8), several types of SLCN are persistent, lifelong or have impacts which affect a young person throughout their childhood and into adulthood. As pupils move into secondary school and beyond, their needs will change in line with the changes in setting, delivery and expectations on them. It is therefore vital we consider how we can work with pupils to prepare them for these changes and equip them with skills that they can carry through past the education years. This will include co-producing goals and working with the pupils themselves to help them to understand their own needs and identify and manage situations that may be challenging for them. As in previous chapters, several of the strategies we will discuss below are useful to consider for all pupils, not just those with SLCN.

STARTING POINTS

- What are some of the key differences between secondary and further education compared to primary education?
- How might some of these differences impact pupils with SLCN?
- What strategies are you already using in your teaching practice to make adaptations for older pupils with SLCN?

SLCN in the secondary school years

The transition to secondary school can be a stressful and challenging time for any pupil (Riglin et al., 2013) but can pose some specific difficulties for those pupils with SLCN (Gough Kenyon et al., 2020). The changes between primary and secondary education are numerous and represent differences in the way content is delivered, how pupils access the classroom, and changes within the individual as they grow and develop as learners and people.

As is evident from Table 13.1, pupils with SLCN are more likely to have difficulties accessing secondary education beyond those we would expect any child transitioning to experience. This is reflected in the outcomes for pupils at the end of secondary schooling and beyond – pupils with Developmental Language Disorder (DLD) (see Chapter 7), for example, do not perform as well as their peers at GCSE (Dubois et al., 2020). This is perhaps unsurprising considering the correlation between language ability and success at GCSE level (Spencer et al., 2017).

When considering how we address these needs for pupils, it is vital that we consider several factors in the instruction we deliver or the adaptations we make. We first want to consider how functional the goals we are setting are, or how useful they will be to the pupil in their day-to-day activities. We must also consider if the skills we are providing

Table 13.1 A summary of key differences between primary and secondary settings and the potential impact for pupils with SLCN

Difference in setting	Potential impact on pupil with SLCN
Size – secondary schools are often much larger than primary schools.	Pupils with SLCN and other types of SEN may find it difficult to navigate the geography of a larger school without support and have difficulty creating an internal 'map' of the school.
Multiple classrooms – a significant change in how lessons are delivered with time spent with multiple subjects in multiple classrooms.	Pupils with SLCN may have difficulties with consolidating learning between classes when required to switch quickly between topics. Practically, an individual with SLCN may find it difficult to access their timetable.
Multiple teachers – a pupil can expect to encounter several different teachers throughout the school day.	There may be fewer opportunities for individual staff members to get to know pupils well enough to identify they are having difficulties. And busy staff members may find it difficult to familiarise themselves or implement adjustments needed for individual pupils.
Expectations – the expectations on learners to independently manage their own time and learning can be challenging.	Pupils who have required a lot of scaffolding and support at primary may not enter secondary school with the skills to manage their own learning or identify when they need support.

(Continued)

Table 13.1 *(Continued)*

Difference in setting	Potential impact on pupil with SLCN
Language – the language of learning becomes more complicated, and more concepts are introduced.	Pupils with SLCN can have difficulties with acquiring new vocabulary and retrieving taught vocabulary, particularly when it is specific to a certain topic. They may also find it difficult to understand non-literal language or idioms, and to process large chunks of information or instruction in one go.
Demands – the increased cognitive load of secondary school, coupled with increasingly complicated peer relationships can be stressful.	Pupils with SLCN can find it hard to maintain peer relationships as their peers' language use becomes more complex. They are at higher risk of social stress (Wadman et al., 2011). They may find it more difficult to manage the challenges of the educational workload. Pupils with SLCN are at higher risk of emotional and behavioural problems compared to their peers (Yew and O'Kearney, 2013).

instruction for are generalisable, that they can be applied to wider contexts and situations than where the instruction is delivered. It is good to consider, for example, how we can specifically teach science vocabulary around homeostasis in a biology class, but even more effective if we can equip the pupil with strategies that will allow them to acquire and retain new vocabulary in any topic or subject. This is particularly pertinent for young people with SLCN as their ability to generalise learning is often weaker than their peers (Leonard et al., 2007; Collisson et al., 2015) which means it is far more difficult for them to link concepts and experiences they know to novel ones.

Transition to secondary school

A successful start to secondary school can lay the foundations for success for the years to follow. Whilst the definition of a successful transition can vary between teaching staff, pupils, and parents and carers, the literature indicates there are some common themes of what can make an effective transition.

The quality of communication is often cited in the literature as a factor in the success of a transition (Bagnall et al., 2020). This includes communication between the departing primary and receiving secondary schools, communication between the school and parents, and acknowledging that some of the burden of communicating relevant information to parents now rests on the pupil. The use of materials to facilitate communication between home and school such as home-school books can be an effective strategy to ensure students with SLCN are able to share appropriate information (Cromwell and Fox, 2023). Technological advances mean that the traditional pen and paper book can often be replaced or supplemented with digital communications to enhance communication between home and school.

The opportunity to have multiple chances to visit the school before full transition at the start of the academic year is also highly valued by parents of children with SEND and by pupils (Cromwell and Fox, 2023). The most effective use of this time will also include opportunities to meet key support staff such as teaching assistants which can allay some of the anxiety for the pupil and their parent/carer around leaving the support systems at primary (Maras and Aveling, 2006).

Ideal communication will also involve support services that have been or remain involved in the pupil's care (Maras and Aveling, 2006). Whilst there can be challenges with establishing where this support exists and who holds responsibility for it, health services such as speech and language therapists should be invited to transition meetings for continuity of care and to input into the support needs of the pupil. Practically, this may involve asking the primary school or the parent/carer for this contact information.

ⓘ CRITICAL QUESTIONS

- What measures do you already put in place to support transition for pupils with SLCN?
- How do you effectively communicate between home and school? Have you encountered any barriers to effective communication?

GUIDANCE FOR ADAPTIVE TEACHING

Several strategies and interventions previously detailed in earlier chapters can be adapted – or are already suitable – to meet the needs of older children and young people with SLCN:

- The strategies outlined in Chapter 2 around adapting the environment to encourage attention and checking understanding are as relevant to secondary school pupils as they are for primary school pupils.
- *Language for Behaviour and Emotions* (Branagan et al., 2021) as detailed in Chapter 4, contains scenarios appropriate for pupils up to age 14 to assess and develop their emotional vocabulary and emotional regulation.
- Vocabulary continues to develop throughout the teenage years and into early adulthood and as such, the vocabulary teaching strategies outlined in Chapter 7 are useful tools to consider in the classroom for teaching topic specific vocabulary.
- Likewise, the guidance for developing literacy alongside spoken language in Chapter 8 can be applied to older children and adolescents. Which is particularly important considering over 120,000 pupils enter secondary school with below expected reading levels (Education Endowment Foundation, 2021).
- The content in Chapter 11 provides a framework for thinking about the whole classroom and its role in supporting pupils with SEMH.

Self-advocacy and workplace skills for pupils with SLCN

A key part of preparation for adulthood is equipping young people with the skills to thrive in the workplace. This includes the ability to self-advocate for support and reasonable adjustments under the Equality Act (2010). This is particularly true considering that employers' knowledge and awareness of SLCN (such as DLD) is much lower compared to other types of learning needs such as autism and dyslexia (de Lemos et al., 2022).

Before being able to advocate for themselves, it is of course key that pupils understand their own needs. This can be inherently difficult for pupils with language difficulties and they may have little or unrealistic insight into their own challenges (Norbury et al., 2016). Guiding a pupil to understand their needs should be bespoke for the individual and be a collaborative process which facilitates the individual to recognise areas of strength and difficulty.

There are published interventions available for supporting pupils with, for example, DLD, to recognise the differences to their peers, understand the implications of their diagnosis, and work towards being able to advocate for themselves and appreciate what adjustments support them best. For example, *DLD and Me* (Sowerbutts and Finer, 2019) is a 12-week intervention programme which aims to help children and young people with DLD understand their strengths and needs. It provides four broad sections that:

- help the young person to talk about and describe themselves;
- discuss what we mean by communication and language in a way that is accessible to the young person;
- helps them to understand their specific diagnosis;
- allows them to develop and identify strategies and begin to self-advocate.

Some of these strategies for use by the young person and adults around them include:

- Making suggestions of approaches that may be useful and allowing the pupil to use their own experiences and knowledge to decide which to adopt. This considers input from the pupil and allows them to make decisions based on ease of use and utility.
- Giving the pupil the language to discuss and disclose their diagnosis to others. A diagnosis is a deeply personal experience, and care should be taken to ensure a pupil can share it in their own words, rather than presenting a stock script.
- Explaining the diagnosis in a way that is accessible to the pupil. This might include using simple language or supporting the communication of the diagnosis using visuals or alternative media such as video or audio. The diagnosis should have been explained at the time it was given, but it may be necessary to revisit this, so the pupil understands what it means in the moment, for example, if it was given several years prior – what does it mean now that they are at secondary school?

Whilst the aforementioned skills are very relevant to pupils' secondary school lives, they also have direct application to preparing pupils for the workplace. There are numerous initiatives nationally to support pupils with SEND to be ready for the working world, but few specifically for pupils with SLCN. *Talk for Work* (I CAN, 2022; now 'Speech and Language UK') is a specific intervention for pupils with language difficulties that, like *DLD and Me*, encourages self-advocacy but with a stronger focus on the skills required to move into the workplace. *Talk for Work* supports pupils through a 14-week programme culminating in a presentation to local employers and along the way demonstrates to pupils:

- the value of recognising different communication styles: aggressive, passive, assertive
- how to recognise when a breakdown in communication has occurred with colleagues/ employers and what exactly might have led to this;
- what skills are valued by employers and how these might differ from pupils' expectations.

Transition to further education/employment

As their time in secondary school education comes to an end, pupils with SEND place high value on independent living skills and autonomy in their own decision-making similar to their peers (Howell, 2023). Face-to-face careers and job coaching with involvement from stakeholders, such as parents or carers, have been demonstrated to be the most effective way of supporting pupils with SEND into employment and creating relationships with employers that are predictors of career success (Hanson et al., 2017). Opportunities for hands-on learning experiences such as volunteering or work placements tend to be the most successful, and young people with SLCN will benefit from the opportunity to have concrete learning experiences that help them learn exactly what will be expected of them in the work environment (Malkani, 2021).

The factors involved in successfully transitioning from secondary school to a further education institution such as a sixth form college share similarities with the transition from primary to secondary school. The key difference is the increased level of involvement from the pupil themselves. Successfully equipping the pupil with skills to recognise and manage their own needs will allow greater opportunities for them to be an active participant in transition planning for their next steps after secondary school.

Further and higher education

Whilst identification of underlying SLCN is improving in a way that correlates with increased awareness, there is still a huge amount of unidentified SLCN in older children and young adults (Clegg et al., 2021). It may be surprising for some to consider that identification of needs such as DLD might not happen until an individual reaches further or higher education, but it is entirely possible for somebody to mask their needs until they meet the demands of this level of education. Masking can be used by young people with DLD for several reasons, including to protect the individual from perceived loss of social status or friendships, or because of the perceived vulnerability of letting people know about their communication difficulty (Hobson and Lee, 2023). It is therefore incumbent on educators at this level to have some awareness of what signs may indicate unidentified SLCN. Signposting to resources to support this can be found at the end of this chapter.

The types of accommodations made by higher education institutions, such as allowing extra time in exams and taking exams in a smaller classroom, are not sufficiently tailored to the needs of individuals with SLCN (Weis et al., 2016). The specific nature of SLCN such as DLD means that specific accommodations are required over more general ones. For example, having access to recordings of lectures and a list of topic-specific vocabulary can address the verbal memory deficits and word learning difficulties a learner with DLD might experience (Del Tufo and Earle, 2020). As previously mentioned, involving the individual learner in decision-making about accommodations is vital to ensuring their needs are met appropriately.

CASE STUDY

Andrea, secondary school SENCo and teacher of English and maths

In January of 2020, I began a new role in an outstanding secondary school as a special educational needs coordinator. I initially trained as a primary teacher – but found myself working in a large secondary school with students that had difficulty accessing mainstream education. My school had a diverse cohort from disadvantaged backgrounds – many of our students qualifying for free school meals.

Fast forward to the next academic year when Charlie, a year 10 student with an EHCP and diagnosis of autism, was refusing to enter the school or leave his mum's car each morning. He would be biting his mother, fighting off staff and presenting as anxious and overwhelmed at the prospect of stepping through the school doors. The trouble was we knew that once Charlie made his way into school he was able to access the lessons and presented as settled. This disconnect between home and school was baffling and caused some friction between school and family. We could not continue with Charlie having this level of distress each morning only to have him mask these feelings when finally crossing the threshold.

Seeking advice from the local authority specialist teachers, they suggested helping Charlie to understand the reasoning behind school, as often students with barriers to communication and interaction will not intrinsically see the bigger picture. We started by gathering Charlie's views and explored what he wanted to do in his future; he had never thought beyond surviving year 11. Charlie explained that he wanted to work in a practical, hands-on way and could see himself doing an apprenticeship so he didn't care about school. This allowed us to explore how we could support him in what he saw as his future. We created a bespoke programme of 'work experience' in school with adults that he knew and who understood him. He began a weekly programme of 1:1 with one of our site managers learning to do hands-on jobs around the school, he also had one session a week working in reception and was trained to be a peer mentor for students in year 7 that struggled with their experience in school.

To accommodate this, we needed to reduce his GCSE offer – a challenge as we want to ensure a broad and balanced curriculum offer for all our SEND learners – but also give Charlie a tailored programme that would motivate him to attend school and have success in his chosen subjects. We needed to show to the leadership team and governing board that this choice would actually expand his life chances and increase his attendance and likelihood of achieving his chosen GCSEs. Luckily, they trusted the process and Charlie was able increase his attendance, he had fewer 'meltdowns' in school, and he achieved passing grades in his GCSEs (including a four in maths and English). He went on to attend college and continued to do work experience in a different school in the Academy Trust.

ⓘ Critical questions

- What supports are in place in your school for pupils like Charlie?
- Are there similar instances of creative and flexible planning occurring in your school?
- Andrea describes Charlie as not thinking of "surviving beyond year 11"; how can we identify and support young people who are only focused on surviving and help them to thrive instead?

SPOTLIGHT ON EMERGING DEBATES

Young people's relationship with technology is very different from that of previous generations, and young people with SLCN are no different from their peers in this regard. There is understandable apprehension around pupils' use of technology, including the dependence on internet usage and social media (Aziz et al., 2024), the potential for cyberbullying and gender-based victimisation (Afrouz and Vassos, 2024), as well as the potential implications on the mental health of young people who spend increasing time online (Shen et al., 2024). However, as digital literacy becomes ever more vital to accessing the world, there are promising developments in the use of technology to support young people with SLCN. This includes the use of speech-to-text to mediate written language difficulties (Matre and Cameron, 2024), accessing learning through virtual and augmented reality (Bailey et al., 2022), and a supportive effect of social media in young people with social anxiety (Angelini and Gini, 2024). Technology is proving to be a key resource in education and onwards in the workplace, so it is incumbent on educators to be open-minded and explore advantages of technological supports.

CHAPTER SUMMARY

Young people with SLCN will often experience difficulties that persist through later childhood/adolescence into adulthood. It is vital that education staff at every level understand the types of needs and adjustments relevant to this group of pupils. We can achieve this through an awareness of the evidence base and most importantly by listening to the individual and facilitating them to be able to communicate their own needs and accommodations.

Further reading/resources

'DLD and me' provide resources for educators and families of young people with DLD at https://www.dldandme.org/

AFASIC are a charity who support children and young people with SLCN and offer transition to secondary school courses https://www.afasic.org.uk/

Speech and Language UK have guidance for identifying SLCN in young people from early years to young adulthood. https://speechandlanguage.org.uk/

References

Afrouz, R and Vassos, S (2024) Adolescents' experiences of cyber-dating abuse and the pattern of abuse through technology, a scoping review. *Trauma, Violence, & Abuse*, 25(4): 2814–2828.

Angelini, F and Gini, G (2024) Differences in perceived online communication and disclosing e-motions among adolescents and young adults: The role of specific social media features and social anxiety. *Journal of Adolescence*, 96(3): 512–525.

Aziz, M, Chemnad, K, Al-Harahsheh, S, Abdelmoneium, A O, Bagdady, A, Hassan, D A, and Ali, R (2024) The influence of adolescents essential and non-essential use of technology and Internet addiction on their physical and mental fatigues. *Scientific Reports*, 14(1): 1745.

Bagnall, C L, Skipper, Y, and Fox, C L (2020) 'You're in this world now': Students', teachers', and parents' experiences of school transition and how they feel it can be improved. *British Journal of Educational Psychology*, 90(1): 206–226.

Bailey, B, Bryant, L, and Hemsley, B (2022) Virtual reality and augmented reality for children, adolescents, and adults with communication disability and neurodevelopmental disorders: A systematic review. *Review Journal of Autism and Developmental Disorders*, 9(2): 160–183.

Branagan, A, Cross, M, and Parsons, S (2021) *Language for Behaviour and Emotions: A Practical Guide to Working with Children and Young People*. 1st edition. [Online]. Oxford: Routledge.

Clegg, J, Crawford, E, Spencer, S, and Matthews, D (2021) Developmental Language Disorder (DLD) in young people leaving care in England: A study profiling the language, literacy and communication abilities of young people transitioning from care to independence. *International Journal of Environmental Research and Public Health*, 18(8): 4107.

Collisson, B A, Grela, B, Spaulding, T, Rueckl, J G, and Magnuson, J S (2015) Individual differences in the shape bias in preschool children with specific language impairment and typical language development: Theoretical and clinical implications. *Developmental Science*, 18(3): 373–388.

Cromwell, H and Fox, C (2023) School transition and SEND: Investigating parental accounts of their child's primary to secondary school transition experience through the use of Mumsnet data. *Psychology of Education Review*, 47(2): 49–56.

de Lemos, C, Kranios, A, Beauchamp-Whitworth, R, Chandwani, A, Gilbert, N, Holmes, A, Pender, A, Whitehouse, C, and Botting, N (2022) Awareness of developmental language disorder amongst workplace managers. *Journal of Communication Disorders*, 95: 106165.

Del Tufo, S N and Earle, F S (2020) Skill profiles of college students with a history of developmental language disorder and developmental dyslexia. *Journal of Learning Disabilities*, 53(3): 228–240.

Dubois, P, St-Pierre, M C, Desmarais, C, and Guay, F (2020) Young adults with developmental language disorder: A systematic review of education, employment, and independent living outcomes. *Journal of Speech, Language, and Hearing Research*, 63(11): 3786–3800.

Education Endowment Foundation (2021) *Improving literacy in secondary schools. Guidance report*. Available at: https://educationendowmentfoundation.org.uk/education-evidence/guidance-reports/literacy-ks3-ks4 (Accessed: 22nd of January 2025).

Equality and Human Rights Commission. (2010). Equality Act 2010 Employment Statutory Code of Practice.

Gough Kenyon, S M, Lucas, R M, and Palikara, O (2020) Expectations of the transition to secondary school in children with developmental language disorder and low language ability. *British Journal of Educational Psychology*, 90(2): 249–265.

Hanson, J, Codina, G, and Neary, S (2017) *Transition programmes for young adults with SEND*. [online]. Available at: https://www.careersandenterprise.co.uk/media/xqhliamz/what-works-report-transition-send.pdf (accessed 23rd January 2025).

Hobson, H M and Lee, A (2023) Camouflaging in developmental language disorder: The views of speech and language pathologists and parents. *Communication Disorders Quarterly*, 44(4): 247–256.

Howell, S (2023) *Exploring the perspectives of young people with SEND during the transition out of further education: a study using Q-Methodology* (Doctoral dissertation, University of East Anglia). Available at: Microsoft Word - 2022 Howell, S EdPsyD.docx (https://ueaeprints.uea.ac.uk/id/eprint/91694/1/2023HowellSREdPsyD.pdf) (accessed 24 February 2025).

I CAN (2022). *Talk for Work*. London: I CAN.

Leonard, L B, Davis, J, and Deevy, P (2007) Phonotactic probability and past tense use by children with specific language impairment and their typically developing peers. *Clinical Linguistics & Phonetics*, 21(10): 747–758.

Malkani, R (2021) Investigating the opportunities provided for young adults with special education needs and disabilities (SEND) to prepare for adulthood in a city in England. *Support for Learning*, 36(2): 238–257.

Maras, P and Aveling, E L (2006) Students with special educational needs: Transitions from primary to secondary school. *British Journal of Special Education*, 33(4): 196–203.

Matre, M E and Cameron, D L (2024) A scoping review on the use of speech-to-text technology for adolescents with learning difficulties in secondary education. *Disability and Rehabilitation: Assistive Technology*, 19(3): 1103–1116.

Norbury, C F, Gooch, D, Wray, C, Baird, G, Charman, T, Simonoff, E, Vamvakas, G, and Pickles, A (2016) The impact of nonverbal ability on prevalence and clinical presentation of language disorder: Evidence from a population study. *Journal of child psychology and psychiatry*, 57(11): 1247–1257.

Riglin, L, Frederickson, N, Shelton, K H, and Rice, F (2013) A longitudinal study of psychological functioning and academic attainment at the transition to secondary school. *Journal of Adolescence*, 36(3): 507–517.

Shen, C, Smith, R B, Heller, J, Spiers, A D, Thompson, R, Ward, H, Roiser, J P, Nicholls, D, and Toledano, M B (2024) Depression and anxiety in adolescents during the COVID-19 pandemic in relation to the use of digital technologies: Longitudinal cohort study. *Journal of Medical Internet Research*, 26: e45114.

Sowerbutts, A and Finer, A (2019) *DLD and Me: Supporting Children and Young People with Developmental Language Disorder*. London: Routledge.

Spencer, S, Clegg, J, Stackhouse, J, and Rush, R (2017) Contribution of spoken language and socio-economic background to adolescents' educational achievement at age 16 years. *International Journal of Language and Communication Disorders*, 52(2): 184–196.

Wadman, R, Durkin, K and Conti-Ramsden, G, (2011) Social stress in young people with specific language impairment. *Journal of adolescence*, 34(3), pp.421–431.

Weis, R, Dean, E L, and Osborne, K J (2016) Accommodation decision making for post-secondary students with learning disabilities: Individually tailored or one size fits all?. *Journal of Learning Disabilities*, 49(5): 484–498.

Yew, S G K and O'Kearney, R, (2013) Emotional and behavioural outcomes later in childhood and adolescence for children with specific language impairments: Metaanalyses of controlled prospective studies. *Journal of child psychology and psychiatry*, 54(5), pp. 516–524.

14 Creating inclusive environments that maximise functional speech, language and communication skills

Niki Stokes and Lorraine Bamblett

- Universal approaches to use across the key stages
- Communication friendly classrooms
- Creating inclusive environments
- Neuroaffirming practice
- Making environments accessible

🎯 CHAPTER OBJECTIVES

This chapter brings together strategies, ideas and resources for SLCN from the other chapters and:

- outlines the key barriers to learning faced by pupils within the range of SLCN;
- suggests ways to overcome these barriers;
- signposts research, strategies, programmes and interventions that can be further consulted or employed to enhance inclusivity for pupils with SLCN in mainstream classrooms.

Introduction

It is acknowledged that there is a SEND crisis in UK schools (Hayes, 2025) and the majority of teachers teach children with additional needs daily. Two from every class of 30 pupils will have Developmental Language Disorder (DLD) (Norbury et al., 2016) and up to around three may have (or have overcome) speech sound disorders (Eadie et al., 2015). Some studies estimate that 10% of all children are experiencing SLCN, but in areas of significant disadvantage this can rise to 50–55% at school entry (Gascoigne, 2024).

The drive towards meeting the ambitions of the Salamanca Statement (UNESCO, 1994) that systems and programmes within education should be designed to take account of the wide diversity of children with SEND and that all children should have access to provision catered for these needs is failing. The implications of this are huge. Our national pedagogy should include the embedded aim to be child-centred and meet the needs of **all** *within the same classes, within the same schools*. We are not at that point yet. Whilst these are high-level and strategic issues that need further consideration, this chapter outlines some practical strategies that can be taken at teacher level to try and improve the environment and pedagogy in our mainstream classes, to support pupils with SLCN.

🚩 STARTING POINTS

- How do you identify SLCN in your cohorts?
- How do you incorporate advice and strategies suggested by outside agencies, e.g. SaLTs, autism outreach, educational psychologists, etc.?
- What barriers to this exist?

Who needs inclusive environments anyway?

A study published in Australia (Glasby et al., 2022) suggested that whilst most teachers believed they were good at identifying speech and language difficulties, their demonstrated capability and understanding of SLCN was mismatched, there was a demonstrated lack of knowledge surrounding specific speech, language and communication needs and how these were identified. This led to difficulties in both implementing strategies for successful inclusion of pupils and impacting teacher's ability to evaluate their effectiveness. Dockrell et al. (2017) compared the views and understanding of education professionals and of SaLTs about SLCN and found that there was less familiarity with terminology used to describe speech difficulties and often no clear understanding between language and speech. This was linked to the lack of coverage of SLCN for trainee teachers and identification of a large gap in training.

The SEND Code of Practice secures the general presumption in mainstream education law in relation to decisions about where children and young people with SEND should be educated (DfE and DoH, 2015). The presumption is that all teachers are teachers of SEND. But, without good understanding of the impacts of SLCN on pupils' learning, it is almost impossible to meet the expectations of pupils, parents, SaLTs, school leaders and school inspection regimes.

Glasby et al. (2022) highlight the lack of understanding that DLD (see Chapter 7), like other neurodivergences, is a lifelong condition and not just a passing difficulty that may resolve over time. This is true of a great many learning differences. Language, argues Glasby et al. (2022), is central to pedagogy and critical to the learning process; this is why strategies that work well for one learning or language need may also be successful for another. Whether the underlying reason the pupil has not understood is that they cannot pay attention to a speaker within a busy classroom environment (see Chapter 2), that their working memory is overloaded, or for another reason entirely, presenting the information in a more accessible way will help. This links to previous chapters (especially 4 and 11) which explore the relationship between SLCN and behaviour.

Accessible pedagogies can support a whole raft of learning differences, overcoming the impacts of SLCN through universal principles, reasonable adjustments, and adaptive teaching: teachers adjusting their practice rather than trying to adjust the pupils. During times when budget constraints, pressures on schools and the SEND system are daily news headlines, being able to accommodate pupils through inclusive practice with all of them in the same classrooms, in the same schools rather than in a little room down the corridor with a teaching assistant (TA) isn't just preferable – it is the *only and expected* way under-resourced teachers can 'manage' their SEND pupils. Rozsahegyi and Lambert (2025) also consider how to balance the two differing agendas of inclusion and raising academic standards and how these may exist side by side. They argue for systemic change both in values and flexibility of provision and the environment so as to accommodate for the specific needs of every child in the classroom, whether they have SLCN, SEND or none of the above.

So, how can this be achieved? Much has been written about the accessible environment and, within England, the drive for Quality First Teaching (QFT) is strong. "A significant proportion of… needs … in the mainstream classroom can be met through High Quality Teaching. This means removing barriers to learning, getting to know and understand individual learners and… bringing the graduated approach to life." (NASEN, 2024).

Barriers to creating an inclusive classroom are multiple: training, resourcing, support from school leaders and a National Curriculum that requires pupils to study their year group's set work regardless of attainment. This requirement to follow the curriculum that matches a child's age is contrary to Vygotsky's theory of proximal development (see Chapter 3), as often it means that children are expected to complete tasks that are within the zone of 'can't do even with guidance'; these expectations are often asked of the child to complete with no support at all and so the child experiences failure. As educators we need to understand each child's capacity for learning, both independently and with support so we can plan activities, strategies and target support for all of the children within our classroom.

So, what strategies can easily be incorporated into **every** classroom, easily and without additional workload?

The accessible environment

Quality First Teaching (QFT) should always be the focus of the universal approach of intervention that sits within the three-tiered model of waves of intervention (universal – targeted – specialist). Robust planning of accessible lessons, effective pedagogical choices and well-considered assessment for learning are key within this approach and will help a school or setting to meet the learning needs of all its children.

Creating an accessible environment is the starting point and should be considered before planning of strategies and lessons takes place. Careful consideration to the environment should also mean that fewer children present with difficulties, because the reasonable adjustments are *already being made* within the classroom due to these environmental changes.

In terms of environmental support, a quick reminder of Maslow's hierarchy of needs (Figure 14.1) highlights that children's physiological needs must be met first. Most schools provide access to water, offer breakfast to hungry children, and ensure adequate heating and cooling systems in classrooms. However, many pupils have other physiological needs, for example, Sensory Processing Disorder (SPD) is often linked to autism and ADHD – which often overlap with SLCN (Reebye and Stalker, 2007). It is also estimated that SPD is under-reported, as children who 'cope' with sensory differences may not be identified – and that up to 16% of all children may have some degree of difficulty in this area (Star Institute, 2024). We have seen pupils dysregulated by sensory need, anxiety and emotional distress operating right at the bottom of the hierarchy of needs. This level of dysregulation inevitably leads to the disruption – and sometimes abandonment – of the lesson for all pupils.

Both feelings of safety and a sense of belonging can be compromised by an environment that is not in tune with a child's sensory needs. Social skills are a big part of social identity and connectedness, with communication a huge part of how these are gained. Being in an environment where there is no support to manage any uncomfortable feelings is also not inclusive.

Another key difficulty that warrants adapted environment considerations are children and young people (CYP) who find it difficult to block out background noise or focus on important

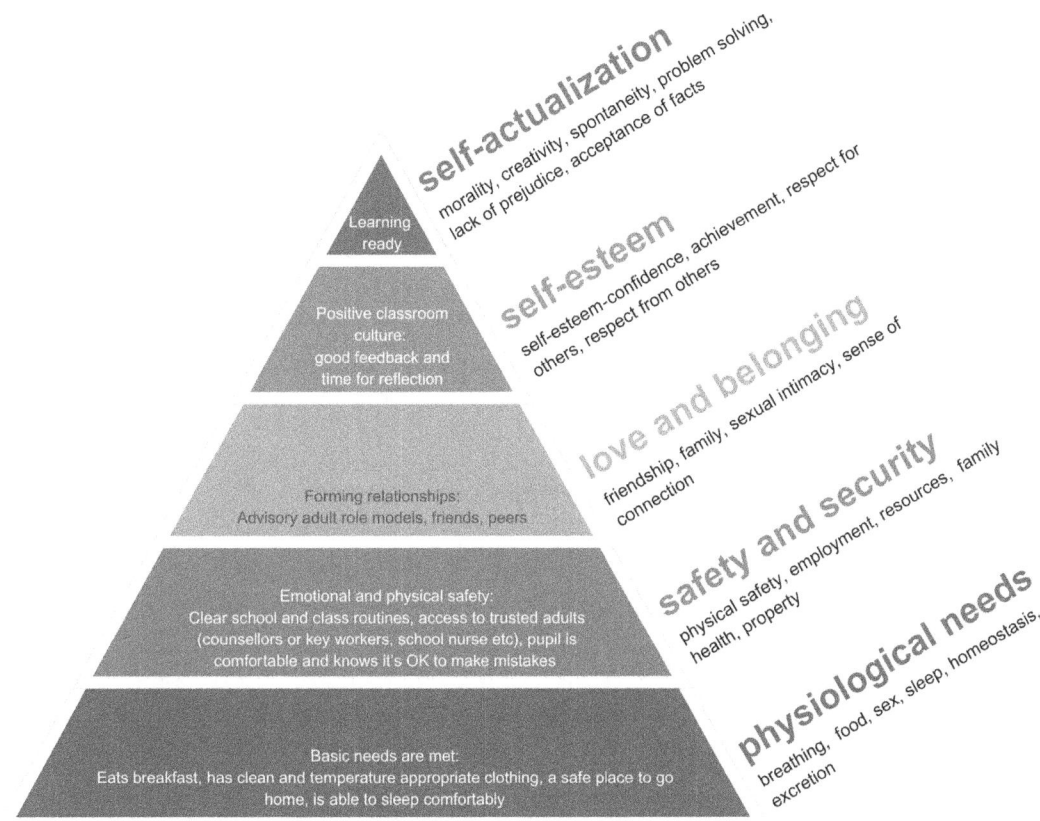

Figure 14.1 Adapted from Maslow's hierarchy of needs (Maslow, 1943)

sounds and can be a key feature of Auditory Processing Disorder (see Chapter 2) and DLD. Quiet classrooms can really support children here – and it is worth reflecting that their needs can be at odds with the standard, child-initiated, free-flow set-up in many EYFS classrooms. This means they are starting school in an environment that does not support their progress and is likely to mean they start KS1 already significantly behind their peers.

This means that a pupil might need reasonable adjustments, such as movement breaks, sensory snacks, noise reduction headphones, chewy or fidget toys, adaptive furniture (such as wobble stools or standing desks), or privacy screens around their work area to block out visual distractions. They may also need a seating plan that acknowledges difficulties with the scent of nearby kitchens or toilets, strongly scented clothes or perfumes, and the use of scented oils to calm or invigorate classrooms. Pupils may need to negotiate changes to uniform, such as understanding that labels can be cut out or that a child wears a tight base layer under their uniform to avoid issues with textures.

Advice on what may help an individual child or classroom environment can be sought from an occupational therapist, accessed via your Special Educational Needs (and Disabilities) Co-ordinator (SENCo/SENDCo) (in collaboration with parents) or through teacher sensory screening, such as this useful one from Affect Autism:

https://affectautism.com/wp-content/uploads/2016/05/Sensory-Problems-Assessment-Questionnaire-2010.pdf [accessed 4 April 2025].

Whatever the barrier, removing the source of the stress is always the best remedy, and understanding the pupil's stressors will guide mitigation.

Communication friendly classrooms

'Communication Friendly', as defined by the Communication Trust, describes the organisation of physical spaces, the strategies that adults use and the opportunities built into each day for CYP to practise their communication skills. We have considered these areas and included some ideas within each to support teachers to adapt their environment to be more communication friendly.

The CYP may benefit from a physical environment that is/has:

- uncluttered with visual timetables and visual cues;
- clearly labelled equipment storage;
- planned seating arrangements;
- additional resources, such as alternative methods of communication or recording, managed background noise;
- clear and consistent routines.

As you can see, a lot of these strategies are similar to those mentioned within our discussion around the accessible environment for CYP with sensory needs which further demonstrates that with simple adaptations to the classroom, CYP with various SEND will be able to access the classroom more successfully.

Strategies adults can use that are helpful include:

- using visual supports and practical teaching approaches;
- objects of reference – physical items that are used to represent a person, activity, place or idea;
- photos, symbols and video, gesture, pointing, showing and sign-supported English alongside talking, all support understanding;
- emphasising key points and slowing down your own speech gives children time to process instructions or questions and frame their responses (see Chapter 7).

A key challenge with SEND teaching within the mainstream class is that SEND pupils typically benefit from both pre-teaching and over-learning. We recognise that this can be challenging in terms of time, staffing and resources. Integrating possible solutions as an added extra may not be feasible and so the use of a whole school approach, from which all children would benefit, is often the solution.

GUIDANCE FOR ADAPTIVE PLANNING

Derbyshire Sensory Toolkit is a comprehensive and evidence-based online tool developed by a multidisciplinary team to help audit the current surroundings and identify if they are impacting on a pupil, and what mitigation can be undertaken to make the environment more inclusive. The intention is that reasonable adjustments, part of 'quality first teaching', are made by carrying out a sensory audit and implementing universal strategies that support a pupil's sensory needs. The toolkit also directs practitioners to further sources of support if the needs of the pupil are beyond the reach of reasonable adjustments and need more specialist support.

Opportunities to practise communication skills might include (see also Chapter 1):

- oracy, including word play sessions, whole school vocabulary building approaches such as Word Aware, and interventions such as Nuffield Early Language Intervention (NELI);
- talk-partner work throughout the day;
- small group discussions, with adult support to guide roles or provide topics, suggest words and help with sentence structure, etc.;
- role playing gives lots of opportunities to practise using new vocabulary, for example, "Mantle of the Expert" type activities;
- rehearsing oral responses and using writing frames or starter sentences for paragraphs can be very helpful for some pupils.

 ## Specific pedagogical approaches

It is important to work with other professionals involved in a pupil's support. If there is a plan supplied by a SaLT, it might contain suggestions for use in the wider classroom and it will certainly suggest regular activities that should be done within school. If these activities can be built into the general classroom practice in any way, this is helpful. These strategies and ideas often fit into the three waves of intervention mentioned previously. Universal approaches suggested by other professionals should form part of everyday practice within the classroom to ensure that CYP with SLCN are considered within teaching throughout the day, not only when they are part of targeted, small-group work or more specialist one-to-one interventions.

Whilst we do not have space to consider all approaches that can be used within the classroom in any detail, Table 14.1 contains a summary of some key approaches:

One of these strategies is cued articulation (see also Chapter 6). Cued articulation is a system developed by Australian SaLT Jane Passey and widely used by NHS SaLTs. Each of the 44 sounds of English have a corresponding hand sign, and these gestures relate

Table 14.1 Summary of some key universal approaches with links to resources

Universal Approach	Key resources with links
Language Screeners	The Nuffield Language Screen and Intervention https://www.teachneli.org/languagescreen/ Wellcomm Language Screen and Intervention https://www.gl-assessment.co.uk/assessments/products/wellcomm/ Language Link screening packages for children aged 3–14. https://speechandlanguage.link/whole-school-approach/
Vocabulary	Word Aware approach https://thinkingtalking.co.uk/word-aware/ Enriching vocabulary in Secondary Schools https://www.taylorfrancis.com/books/mono/10.4324/9780429433177/enriching-vocabulary-secondary-schools-victoria-joffe-hilary-lowe Online vocabulary resources from Vocabulary Ninja: https://vocabularyninja.co.uk/product-category/vocabulary/
Sentence Construction	Colourful Semantics https://www.integratedtreatmentservices.co.uk/our-approaches/speech-therapy-approaches/colourful-semantics-2/
Phonological Awareness and Phonics	The Newcastle Intervention for Phonological Awareness and the Newcastle Intervention for Phonological Awareness https://research.ncl.ac.uk/phonologicalawareness/Cued Articulation (see below) https://www.elklan.co.uk/Shop/Cued_Articulation
Visual Supports	Software for schools to add visual support and symbols https://widgitonline.com/en/home
Social Interaction	Lego-based therapy https://legobasedtherapy.org/ Social Thinking Curriculum https://www.socialthinking.com/detective-superflex-series-social-emotional-learning-curriculum
Emotional Regulation	Zones of Regulation https://www.socialthinking.com/zones-of-regulation

to the way the sound is articulated in the mouth. This acts as a reminder to a child struggling with articulation what they need to do with their tongue and lips in order to correct their speech sound. However, it is possible to also incorporate cued articulation into your teaching of phonics. Much as the Jolly Phonics synthetic phonics system has an 'action' for each phoneme, cues for each sound can be taught. This has not been fully evaluated through rigorous research – but anecdotally we introduced cued articulation in a speech and language centre KS1 class some years ago and were extremely surprised to find the children were able to learn the cues much faster than the Jolly Phonics signs. Even better, we found they would refer to the phonics display on the wall and then start doing the cues whilst saying a word to remember how to write the sound, a strategy we had struggled to get them to use when employing the scheme actions. It appeared as if the action being linked to the way they [were being taught to] make the sound helped them to bridge between phoneme and grapheme and to hold the sound in mind whilst running through the written representations. It is possible to incorporate these cues with other validated phonics systems whilst maintaining the fidelity of the programme.

As discussed in Chapter 7, the early years are crucial and identifying difficulties at a young age is helpful as strategies taught as young as possible give children the best chance to achieve their best. There are various language screeners available, e.g. NELI, Wellcomm or Language Link, to identify the children with the weakest vocabulary and comprehension skills. We have provided links to these in the Table 14.1.

⑦ CRITICAL QUESTIONS

- How do you organise the classroom environment to support children with difficulties with speaking, listening, understanding or communicating?
- What reasonable adjustments do you make for sensory needs?
- What universal approaches can you bring into your classroom to include more children with SLCN?
- What further resources and training do you need to develop your practice?

SPOTLIGHT ON EMERGING DEBATES

Our concept of neurodiversity is evolving. We have gone from using 'neurodiverse' to describe mainly autism to understanding that brain architecture differences occur in a range of pupil presentations, including ADHD, DLD, developmental trauma, specific and general learning differences. Further, the introduction of person-centred practices – currently statutory in education, although deployed in different ways in different settings – and particularly pupil/population voice, including adult autistic and other ND advocates, has changed our perspectives on what is the 'right' way to educate neurodiverse cohorts. In some cases, individuals have spoken out against the strategies they were taught, particularly around behaviourist approaches:

The emphasis on things like eye contact or sitting still or not stimming – i.e. self-stimulation such as flapping hands – 'is oriented around trying to create the trappings of the typical child,' says autism self-advocate Ari Ne'eman, without acknowledging the reality that different children have different needs. It can be actively harmful when we teach people from a very early age that the way they act, the way they move is fundamentally wrong.

(Garey, 2024), (https://childmind.org/article/controversy-around-applied-behavior-analysis/)

Approaches to 'treating' autism in SaLT have traditionally been impairment rather than strengths based (Lobsey, 2022). This is because approaches to therapy and education, created by and for neurotypical people, have traditionally taken the view that autistic people need to be 'normalised' (medical approach) rather than recognising, accepting and advocating for neurodivergent people being wired differently, taking an affirmative approach (Pellicano and den Houting, 2022).

Neuro-affirming approaches ask us to accept and adapt our practice to embrace diversity, rather than teach pupils that their differences are unwelcome. They recognise and address the societal barriers neurodiverse people encounter. Neuro-affirming practice is something else that can be at odds with the practice seen in some schools.

Where some programmes written to work on social skills in small groups often promote ideas such as 'eye-contact' and 'sitting still' as desirable, others can seem to promote neurotypical 'flexible thinking' as an aim; these are often anxiety provoking, counterproductive or unrealistic for a neurodivergent CYP. However, with some tweaks, resources such as: Zones of Regulation (where we teach pupils that their intrinsic responses and behaviours are unexpected and give others 'uncomfortable thoughts' about them) and Superflex (where a cast of neurodiverse behaviour 'anti-heroes' fight the neurotypical 'flexible thinking' eponymous superhero) could become more neuro-affirming.

Perhaps a better option is naturalistic, interest-driven opportunities for group working. One example of this is Lego-based therapy, an evidence-based intervention that allows children to experience different group roles, build empathy and learn to work as a team in order to achieve a set task. Learning social scripts by practising, learning from miscommunications and shared success rather than being 'taught the rules' and expected to replicate these in real-life interactions which is what many other programmes designed to work on social communication rely on. Kate Timms describes the use of an adapted version of Lego-based therapy in the following case study.

As the push for inclusive education in mainstream education grows, curriculum approaches for pupils working below the expectations of the National Curriculum – such as Equals, (Imray and Hinchcliffe, 2014) are invaluable. Equals asks practitioners to adapt a multi-tiered curriculum framework in a person-centred way to ensure learners working below the National Curriculum have some agency over how they spend their days – and how stressful that day is for them. Equals can also support a neuro-affirming approach and, once established, can provide a basis for continuing to teach in a truly inclusive way, regardless of academic ability for those pupils with additional SEND.

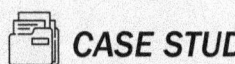 **CASE STUDY**

Kate, SENCo and assistant principal at a primary mainstream school

Pupils with speech, language, and communication needs (SLCN) face significant barriers to learning, struggling with vocabulary, sentence structure and verbal confidence. These challenges impact academic progress, social interactions and classroom engagement. I work in a mainstream primary school in the West Midlands, where communication and interaction is the most prevalent need within our SEN caseload.

Two key pupils with education, health and care plans (EHCPs) had difficulty following multi-step instructions, leading to disengagement and errors. Social communication challenges, such as interpreting social cues and turn-taking, often resulted in frustration, emotional outbursts or withdrawal from learning.

We benefited from speech and language students from Birmingham City University, supported by an SLT lecturer. They provided support and introduced research-backed interventions. One such strategy was Building Together, a play-based programme designed to enhance social competence in children with autism spectrum conditions (ASC) and related difficulties (adapted from Lego-based therapy).

Implemented within Key Stage 2, this intervention aimed to improve communication, collaboration and problem-solving through structured building tasks. One of our dedicated teaching assistants facilitated the intervention, assigning pupils clear roles such as 'builder' and 'instructor' while using visual cue cards to scaffold vocabulary and sentence structures. Instructions were broken into manageable steps and reinforced with gestures or visual aids like Widgit vocabulary mats. The staff member modelled appropriate communication skills, promoting turn-taking and active listening. Pupils were encouraged to verbalise their thought processes, ask for help and describe their actions, fostering problem-solving abilities. As a result, both pupils showed increased engagement, improved communication confidence and better collaboration with peers.

Moving forward, we plan to embed structured social communication interventions like Building Together into our curriculum. Staff will receive additional training to ensure consistency in supporting pupils with SLCN. We also aim to expand the intervention from small groups to whole-class activities, promoting inclusivity and peer collaboration.

This experience highlights the value of targeted interventions for pupils with SLCN. Structured, play-based activities can significantly enhance communication, social interaction and confidence, benefiting both pupils and the wider classroom environment. By fostering explicit support in social communication, we can create inclusive classrooms that improve engagement and overall educational outcomes.

ⓘ Critical questions

- Are there children with social communication, receptive language and expressive language challenges in your classroom?
- Could your children benefit from a structured environment to practice sentence use, initiating and maintaining a conversation for a joint goal?
- Is there an opportunity for a lunchtime or after school Lego club that children could sign up for?

📝 CHAPTER SUMMARY

Creating inclusive, communication friendly spaces is essential for supporting children with SLCN across all school environments. These environments are a key part of the universal approach – strategies that benefit all children whilst particularly supporting those with identified needs. A communication friendly setting encourages interaction, reduces anxiety and promotes confidence through visual supports, accessible language and providing opportunities for meaningful dialogue.

As discussed in this chapter, inclusion goes beyond resources or interventions, it is about fostering a school culture where every child feels heard, understood and valued. By embedding inclusive communication strategies into everyday practice, practitioners help ensure that children with SLCN can participate fully and meaningfully in their learning.

Incorporating neuro-affirming practice – approaches that respect and celebrate neurological differences – is also vital. This means recognising diverse communication styles, avoiding a one-size-fits-all model and creating environments where children feel safe to be themselves.

Through a universal, inclusive and neuro-affirming lens, we can build environments that empower all children to thrive, learn and belong.

📖 Further reading/resources

- Free to access, simple and quick checklist to check your classrooms are Communication Friendly: https://speechandlanguage.org.uk/wp-content/uploads/2023/12/communication_friendly_environments_checklist_updated.pdf
- Nationally accredited training for mainstream, special and specialist settings across all key stages on communication friendly settings: Communication https://www.elklan.co.uk/Training/Settings/

- Derbyshire sensory processing needs toolkit designed to support children with sensory needs to reduce or remove the impact on their learning. https://www.localoffer.derbyshire.gov.uk/site-elements/documents/education-and-learning/spn/dcc-spn-toolkit-v13-interactive.pdf

- Whole School SEND Nasen Teacher Handbook developed to support teachers to embed inclusive practice. https://nasen.org.uk/news/teacher-handbook-launched

 References

DfE and DoH (Department for Education and Department of Health and Social Care) (2015) Special educational needs and disability code of practice 0-25 years. Available at: www.gov.uk/government/publications/send-code-of-practice-0-to-25 accessed 26 February 2025).

Dockrell, J, Howell, P, Leung, D. and Fugard, A (2017) Children with speech language and communication needs in England: Challenges for practice. *Frontiers in Education* 2. https://doi.org/10.3389/feduc.2017.00035

Eadie, P, Morgan, A, Ukoumunne, O C, Ttofari Eecen, K, Wake, M, and Reilly, S (2015) Speech sound disorder at 4 years: Prevalence, comorbidities, and predictors in a community cohort of children. *Developmental Medicine & Child Neurology*, 57(6): 578–584.

Garey, J (2024) The Controversy Around ABA - Child Mind Institute [accessed 4 April 2025].

Gascoigne, M (2024) Meeting speech, language and communication needs: A whole-systems, population-based approach. *Paediatrics and Child Health*, 34(7): 201–210.

Glasby, J, Graham, L J, White, S, and Tancredi, H (2022) Do teachers know enough about the characteristics and educational impacts of Development Language Disorder (DLD) to successfully include students with DLD? *Teaching and Teacher Education*, 119: 103868 https://doi.org/10.1016/j.tate.2022.103868

Hayes, D (2025) SEND crisis: Key challenges and five solutions to fix the system. *Children and Young People Now*, 2025(2): 8–9.

Imray, P and Hinchcliffe, V (2014) *Curricula for Teaching Children and Young People with Severe or Profound Learning Difficulties*. London: Routledge.

Lobsey, N (2022) Ableism is Speech Pathology. Available at: https://therapistndc.org/ableism-speech-pathology/

Maslow, A H (1943) A theory of human motivation. *Psychological Review*, 50(4): 370–396.

NASEN (The National Association for Special Educational Needs) (2024) Teacher Handbook: SEND – Embedding inclusive practice. Available at: https://nasen.org.uk/news/teacher-handbook-launched (accessed 26 February 2025).

Norbury, C F, Gooch, D, Wray, C, Baird, G, Charman, T, Simonoff, E, Vamvakas, G, and Pickles, A (2016) The impact of nonverbal ability on prevalence and clinical presentation of language disorder: Evidence from a population study. *Journal of Child Psychology and Psychiatry*, 57(11): 1247–1257.

Pellicano, E and den Houting, J (2022) Annual Research Review: Shifting from 'normal science' to neurodiversity in autism science. *Journal of Child Psychology and Psychiatry*, 63(4): 381–396.

Reebye, P and Stalker, A S (2007) *Understanding Regulation Disorders of Sensory Processing in Children: Management Strategies for Parents and Professionals* (1st ed.). London: Jessica Kingsley Publishers.

Rozsahegyi, T and Lambert, M (2025) Pedagogy, inclusion and the SENCo's role. In Knowler, H, Richards, H, and Brewster, S (eds). *Developing Your Expertise as a SENCo* (pp. 35–46). London: Routledge.

Star Institute (2024) About sensory processing disorder. Available at: https://sensoryhealth.org/ (accessed 4 March 2025).

UNESCO (1994) *The Salamanca Statement and Framework for Action on Special Needs Education*. Salamanca: World Conference on Special Needs Education: Access and Quality.

15 Interprofessional and collaborative working

Sally Philpotts and Alice Murphy

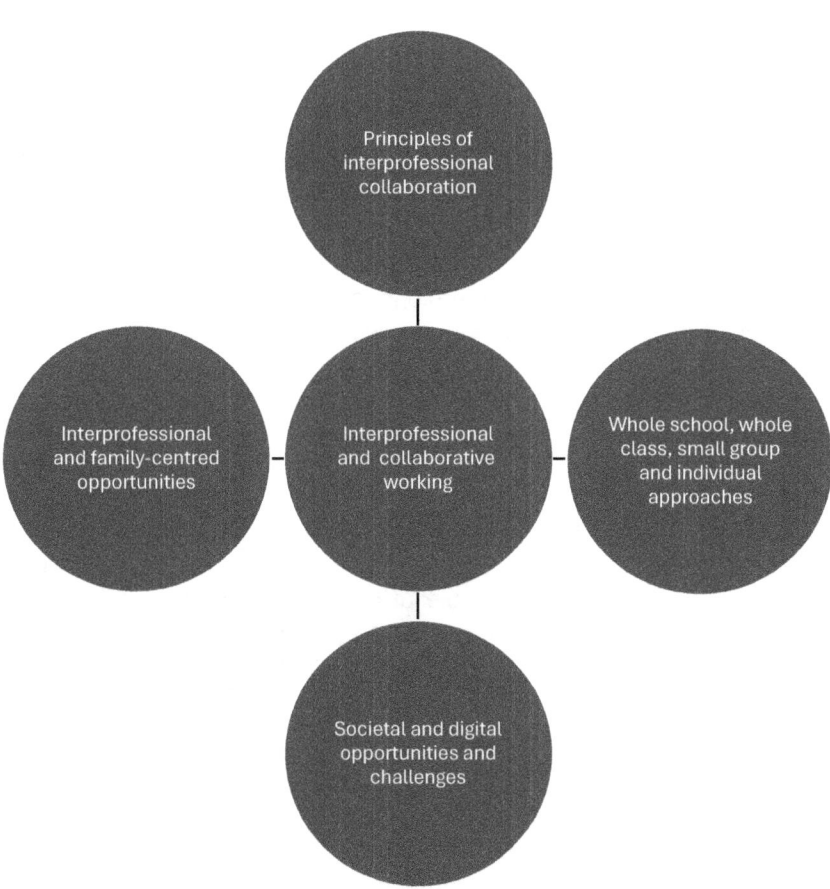

DOI: 10.4324/9781041054986-19

CHAPTER OBJECTIVES

This chapter explores how implementing principles of interprofessional collaboration within inclusive learning environments can impact speech, language and communication (SLC) progress and outcomes. The chapter:

- explores the theories and principles of interprofessional and family-centred collaboration for pupils with speech, language and communication needs (SLCN);
- identifies opportunities available for interprofessional and family-centred approaches;
- identifies differences between whole school, whole class, small group or individual approaches; and
- recognises 21st-century societal and digital opportunities and challenges.

Introduction

Teamwork is integral to schools and to service delivery, be it within classrooms and wider school settings, with parents and carers or with external staff, including educational support departments and other professionals. To support speech, language, and communication needs (SLCN), joined-up assessments, knowledge, goal setting and recommendations can maximise the effectiveness of interventions and the progress of the pupil. Adopting a team-oriented, strategic approach will include considering, examining and implementing strategies at the school-wide, whole class, small group and individual levels. Developing and utilising the knowledge and skills of all concerned enables more efficient support. However, collaborative working will need to become an implicit, embedded part of practice across settings for this to be successful.

Interprofessional and internal staff meetings, training sessions and collaborative approaches such as shared planning (e.g. lesson study) can inspire, inform and engage practitioners in discussions about the role of SLC in shaping and influencing learning. These approaches build confidence integrating these skills into practice. This chapter will therefore focus on the contribution that interprofessional and collaborative working makes to SLC progress and outcomes.

Interprofessional collaboration and family-centred collaboration

STARTING POINTS

- What does interprofessional collaboration mean?
- Who may you collaborate with? What does this look like?

Collaboration involves two or more people, professionals and/or families working together towards a common goal. Friend and Cook (2000) define it as a style of direct interaction between at least two co-equal parties voluntarily engaged in shared decision-making to achieve their common goal.

In the context of collaboration between health services and education, partners can share knowledge, experience, skills and resources to achieve outcomes that are often unattainable when working individually. Unlike either 'cooperation' or 'coordination', collaboration requires deeper integration and mutual engagement through active contributions and the ability to influence each other's work (Castañer and Oliveira, 2020).

Collaborative partners

When forming a collaborative partnership, consider all those involved in supporting the pupil:

- **Pupil**

    Involving the pupil ensures their voice is heard, helping to set shared goals and priorities, which boosts engagement and motivation. This aligns with the SEND Code of Practice (Gov.UK, 2014).

- **Families**

    Whoever the child is living with (birth family, carer or other family figure) offers holistic insight into the pupil and ensures priorities are aligned with cultural beliefs and practices. Their involvement reinforces learning and support outside school.

- **Education professionals**

    Support staff, teachers: Special Educational Needs (and Disabilities) Co-ordinator (SENCo/SENDCo) and school leaders contribute to achieving SLCN outcomes at various levels. They bring firsthand knowledge of the pupil's needs and classroom dynamics, ensuring strategies are implemented practically.

- **Health professionals**

    Speech and language therapists (SaLTs) provide clinical knowledge of the pupil's SLCN. Other health professionals like occupational therapists (OTs), physiotherapists (PTs), paediatricians and child and adolescent mental health services (CAMHS) may be involved, especially when there are overlapping difficulties.

- **Other agencies or support professionals**

    This may include social care, youth justice, charities and other community partners. Local authority members, including educational psychologists and inclusion teams, can also offer additional insights and support.

This streamlined approach ensures all relevant parties contribute effectively to the pupil's progress.

Theories and principles in collaborative practice

> **? CRITICAL QUESTIONS**
>
> Think of a time you have worked with a colleague to support a pupil with SLCN:
>
> - What helped you to achieve positive outcomes for this pupil?
> - Were there any barriers to this?
> - Were there differences in how each person defined a positive outcome? If so, what skills did you use to address this?
> - What do you need to work effectively alongside others when supporting a pupil with SLCN?
> - Does your approach differ when working with professionals versus families?

Within the UK, health and education policies and services focus on collaborative practices within speech and language therapy including family-centred and interprofessional working. With historical acknowledgement of collaborative working within speech and language therapy, there is now an increased focus on the collaboration between education and health professionals with the common goal of improving outcomes for pupils with SLCN (Quigley and Smith, 2021). Alongside this, there is an increased need to identify *how* collaboration can be most effective within modern society. This is particularly relevant when considering current workforce implications, including SaLTs' increasing caseload sizes and the educational implications within teacher recruitment and retention due to increasing workload, with larger class sizes and Ofsted pressures (Gov.UK, 2024). Despite these challenges, the heart of collaborative practice must prioritise the pupil's goals and needs, focusing on how to develop support that is effective and has long-lasting positive impacts.

For effective collaboration between SaLTs, educators and families, there first needs to be an understanding of why this is needed (Mathers, Botting and Moss, 2024). Research demonstrates that both teachers and SaLTs are aware of the high numbers of pupils who require communication support in classrooms and have the shared hope of being able to support pupils with SLCN more effectively (Glover et al., 2015). It is agreed that strong collaborative relationships between allied health professionals and education professionals improves outcomes for pupils with SLCN. These positive outcomes include (but are not exclusive to) increasing access to education, supporting educational outcomes and improving pupil participation within the learning environment (Jeremy, Spandagou and Hinitt, 2024).

Interprofessional collaboration

Interprofessional collaboration involves professionals from different occupations using their professional knowledge and individually learned experiences to work towards the same goal of supporting pupils with SLCN. This complementary transfer of skills has been argued to improve joint problem-solving, leading not only to positive outcomes for pupils but also to identify learning points professionals can use as best practice models; and perhaps most importantly, offer a model of holistic support for pupils with SLCN.

Despite feeling like a common-sense approach, interprofessional collaboration is hard to introduce and maintain effectively when put into practice (Cameron, 2011). Whilst interprofessional collaboration is listed as a core feature of integrated services (Mecrow et al. 2010), systemic barriers such as health and education services working against different frameworks have been identified; resulting in different ways of approaching interactions and goal setting. In addition to this, there are increasing work and caseload demands in both professions, alongside widely reported staffing difficulties meaning effective interprofessional collaboration is not straightforward even with good intentions and a desire to work together. A lack of time to engage in, discuss and embed collaborative practice is highlighted across a range of settings, including mainstream, early years and settings that cater to special educational needs (Hartas, 2004). Alongside this, recent reviews of collaborative working between education and SaLT in UK primary schools highlight the need for improvements, such as gathering the views of TAs (anecdotally described as the unsung heroes that carry out SaLT interventions in schools) and needing a consistent definition of what collaborative practice is (Mathers et al., 2024).

Consistent and effective interprofessional practice will undoubtedly be impacted by these stressors and may reduce the levels of personal and professional support felt by educators and therapists (Wright et al., 2008). Nonetheless, there are recurring themes that increase support and highlight outcome-driven and solution-focused collaborative practice.

An increased understanding of different roles and the boundaries of these will improve outcomes for pupils. A foundation built on shared knowledge and mutual respect supports every voice to be heard and allows a focus on the pupil's needs without hierarchy (Nancarrow et al. 2013). Prioritising these themes and allocating protected time for solution-focused discussions can increase the positive impact of collaborative working. Taking the time to meet with the goal of explicitly building professional relationships also has positive impact on collaborative working (Quigley and Smith, 2021).

Family-centred collaboration

The relationship between teachers and families has been widely researched and was a fundamental development within the SEND Code of Practice (Gov.UK, 2014) based on the Children and Families Act (2014), emphasising the importance of pupil and family involvement in decision-making. Collaboration between school staff and families is a fundamental aspect of the teaching role; this partnership is crucial to enhanced opportunities.

Family-centred collaboration (pupils and families being involved through describing, addressing and prioritising their own needs) is essential to achieving effective collaborative practice. For pupils with SLCN, family-centred collaboration increases the likelihood of improved outcomes for pupils (See and Gorard, 2015).

A common theme within the research into collaboration is that whilst each group – educators and SaLTs, parents and teachers, as well as parents and SaLTs – all have the desire to engage in positive and fulfilling interpersonal relationships, the implementation of collaborative practice is not straightforward and can be challenging (Klatte et al. 2024).

Factors that hinder family-centred collaboration with professionals include parents feeling disempowered, parents' uncertainty about their ability to support their child's educational and SLCN skills, and professional judgements regarding parental competence. Additionally, many challenges encountered in interprofessional collaboration also apply to family-centred approaches, such as:

- **Reduced knowledge sharing**: Whilst educators are the pedagogical experts and SaLTs are the experts in SLCN, pupils and their families are undoubtedly the most knowledgeable about themselves – removing hierarchy and celebrating each person's contribution can influence successful joint planning.
- **Interpersonal relationships**: Building trust and having a shared goal can help to build relationships; empowering families to be active participants by recognising the wider picture and showing respect and empathy.
- **A lack of time and space**: This can be the result of service demands for professionals, but the demands placed on families must be considered. These can include working parents and/or those who have other caring responsibilities.

Settings that have well-established relationships with families can still improve collaboration through reflective practice and joint working. Reflections could include what information is provided within staff training, what is going well and consideration of curriculum demands.

Opportunities available for interprofessional and family-centred approaches

> ⚑ **STARTING POINTS**
> - What collaborative opportunities have you been involved in?
> - How does this help you to support pupils?
> - What impact does this have for your teaching and their learning?

Literature confirms that SaLT support is essential across various educational settings, including early years, mainstream and special schools, colleges and alternative provisions (Gov.UK, 2023). Research highlights the importance and challenges of effective collaboration but applying this knowledge can be overwhelming. To address this, examples of impactful collaboration across educational environments are included. Law et al. (2012)

outlines a framework for speech and language therapy service delivery tiers, similarly identified in the SEND Code of Practice (Gov.UK, 2014).

Whole school

A strategic approach requiring collaboration in a mainstream primary setting following Ofsted feedback which identified improvements to develop a more communication friendly environment.

 CASE STUDY – INTRODUCTION OF WHOLE SCHOOL TASK PLANS

Who?
- TAs, class teachers, SENCo, senior leadership team, SaLT

How?
- SaLT advice requested by SENCo to develop a whole school communication friendly environment.
- Joint audit, led by SaLT and including SENCo plus a school leader with curriculum responsibility.
- Teachers and TAs included within feedback regarding accessibility of information.
- It was found that class expectations and activities were not provided visually/consistently broken down into smaller chunks. Pupils with identified language needs or processing difficulties did not always understand what to do.
- Audit team provided clear feedback for school staff highlighting best practice already in place and three 'quick win' suggestions for improvements.
- Clear rationale for changes provided by all members of the audit team.
- Teachers and TAs introduced to a task plan template created jointly by the audit team (and headteacher approval) at the next training day.
- Working examples of task plans for whole class/individual provided.
- Half-term trial agreed, with opportunities to provide feedback and suggest changes.

Outcome:
- Teacher and TA feedback following trial period provided opportunity to enhance the whole school template and increase staff buy-in.
- TA feedback that pupils with SLCN were more open to using the task plans as they weren't 'different' to their peers and therefore stigma had been reduced.
- Teachers reported that joined-up approaches allowed staff moving classes or teaching a cover lesson to continue implementing communication friendly practice without difficulty.

Whole class

Joined-up working increasing access to education within an alternative provision by developing a whole class emotion regulation programme.

CASE STUDY – WHOLE CLASS EMOTION REGULATION PROGRAMME IN AN ALTERNATIVE PROVISION

Who?

- Class teachers, TAs and SaLT

How?

- Twenty pupils across three classes were screened for SLCN; all identified as having difficulties recognising and identifying their emotions.
- Teaching staff identified that these difficulties impacted pupils' well-being and their ability to access learning.
- Educators shared knowledge regarding the curriculum and individual student background; SaLT shared emotional regulation programme information.
- Jointly agreed outcomes (SaLT, teachers, TAs) encouraged power sharing and removal of hierarchy.
- A solution-focused approach, including identifying clear roles for the planning and delivery of this (in line with individual constraints) helped to build trust and rapport.
- SaLT training provided with half-termly evaluation opportunities for all parties to address concerns or areas to develop.

Outcome:

- Thirteen pupils were able to identify how they were feeling and identify at least one strategy to support them.
- Teachers reported increased length of time pupils were staying in classrooms.
- Educators reported increased confidence in being able to share knowledge with colleagues in other classes.
- SaLT reported increased knowledge of classroom teaching styles, as well as understanding the benefits/constraints of working within a classroom model.
- SaLT used knowledge of classroom model to increase the effectiveness of other SLCN interventions indicating that collaboration has wider reaching implications.

Group work

A family-centred approach to developing attention and listening skills in small groups, offering targeted support in a nursery setting with weekly SaLT input.

CASE STUDY – ATTENTION AND LISTENING GROUPS IN A NURSERY SETTING

Who?

- Early years practitioners (EYP), SaLT and families

How?

- Initial meeting between EYP and SaLT identified attention and listening skills as a concern.
- Agreed outcome within the limited time available: to provide targeted support for a small group of students to develop skills and build staff confidence.
- Target group identified and SMART targets co-produced for each pupil. A complementary skill transfer is the shared knowledge of developmental stages of attention, supplemented by the EYP's early learning goals.
- Joint planning arranged.
- First session was co-produced and delivered together to increase staff confidence – providing valuable insight into how targeted groups can be successful in a nursery.
- Collaboration ensured the intervention was tailored to the individual needs of each pupil and allowed families to continue with activities at home.

Outcome:

- Management of limited time in a demanding setting through solution-focused discussions during each visit.
- EYP reported 'excitement' at carrying the group out and generalised the strategies universally.
- Families felt empowered to continue the interventions at home.
- This example was used as a case study to guide other settings on how to prioritise time and have an impact with limited allocation.

One-to-one

Individual work can take place inside and outside of the classroom. A special school providing supported internships in sixth form required a pupil-centred approach to increase likelihood of a successful outcome of paid employment at the end of the programme.

CASE STUDY – DEVELOPMENT OF APPROPRIATE WORK PLACEMENT SUPPORT BEFORE AND DURING A SUPPORTED INTERNSHIP

Who?
- Pupil, family, SENCo, supported internship placement coordinator, job coach, employer and SaLT

How?
- Placement planning meeting with all to understand pupil aspirations, preferred area of work and concerns about the workplace.
- Pre-placement meeting with all professionals identifying areas where SLCN support may be required, for example, how to request a break or guidance provided visually.
- Jointly developed SLCN outcomes and targets tailored to the work environment.
- SaLT provided training for the job coach and employer explaining SLCN and outlining recommendations to support the pupils' aims and SLC targets.

Outcome:
- Increased employer understanding and empathy leading to wider changes and a willingness to carry out more placements.
- Likert scale pupil ratings showed increased confidence and reduced anxiety about starting placement with new agreed adjustments.
- The functional impact of collaboration meant pupils developed their independence and autonomy.
- Regular opportunities to review progress increased targeted support leading to offers of paid apprenticeships.

Importance of evaluating the impact of collaborative practices

Evaluating collaborative practices is crucial for addressing challenges regarding education access and social inclusion. Disparities in skills, time constraints and communication barriers can hinder effective collaboration, impacting student support. Continuous professional development and adherence to the 'assess, plan, do, review' (APDR) cycles from the SEND Code of Practice (Gov.UK, 2014) increase responsiveness to student needs. This promotes better academic and communication outcomes and strengthens relationships with families through aligning with shared goals.

21st-century opportunities and challenges

Advances in technology, artificial intelligence (AI) and communication tools enhance access and increase collaborative opportunities, improving pupil outcomes. However, they also present challenges, particularly around balancing in-person versus online interactions and ensuring equal access to information.

> **STARTING POINT**
>
> - What digital opportunities are available in your setting?
> - What technology do you currently use?
> - What impact does this have on your workload and SLCN outcomes for pupils?
> - How confident are you when using technology?

Technology significantly enhances access to collaborative opportunities. Software such as TheraPlatform and Provision Map, alongside video conferencing apps including Microsoft Teams, Google Meet and Zoom, facilitate collaboration across social and geographical barriers supporting hard-to-reach stakeholders and underserved areas. Applications including Google Workspace and Microsoft SharePoint facilitate real-time document collaboration, progress tracking and joint planning. A shift to online platforms allows regular, flexible interactions, benefiting schools with limited on-site SaLTs and families unable to attend in-person meetings.

AI tools are starting to revolutionise SLCN identification and support by analysing communication patterns, predicting outcomes and simulating personalised exercises. For instance, Speech and Language Link uses AI to tailor interventions based on individual assessments, making app-based provision cost-effective and convenient, increasing therapy intensity and flexibility.

Applications can also track pupil progress, allowing teachers and SaLTs to access real-time data and tailor interventions, making collaborative planning more efficient. AI tools like Google Translate aid communication with pupils and families who speak different languages, fostering inclusivity and reducing inequalities.

> ### CASE STUDY – USING MICROSOFT SHAREPOINT TO INCREASE COLLABORATIVE PRACTICES IN A MAINSTREAM SECONDARY SETTING
>
> Who?
>
> - SENCo, HLTA (responsibility for interventions), NHS enhanced SaLT (paid service one day per week)
>
> How?
>
> - Immediate access to consent forms, meeting notes, daily intervention records and joint planning.
> - Features such as document libraries and Microsoft OneNote enabling access prior, during and after the day.
>
> Outcome:
>
> - School staff and SaLT reported increased efficiency and reduced workload by using an electronic communication and file sharing system via Microsoft SharePoint.
> - All professionals accessing the same data meant consistent information was shared with families building positive and trusting relationships.

However, technological advancements also pose ethical challenges where access to digital support remains a barrier and risks creating inequalities. Geographical limitations (inconsistent rural internet connectivity) and socio-economic barriers (financial cost of hardware or high-speed internet) may prevent access and potentially reduce effectiveness of collaboration. Ofcom (2023) reports that 98% of higher income households have internet access compared to 84% of lower income households, highlighting the digital divide.

The effectiveness of digital tools depends on users' technological competence and attitude (Leinweber et al. 2023). When planning collaborative practices, consider all parties' willingness, experience and confidence with technology and provide training and support to overcome barriers. Research shows families can be sceptical about teletherapy; professionals should consider family experiences and feelings when discussing it as an option.

Whilst online platforms allow for flexibility, they may not fully replicate the effectiveness of in-person collaboration or support, especially for pupils who require support to develop their attention and listening skills. Specialist one-to-one teletherapy also requires a specific level of attention, which not all pupils with SLCN will have. Anecdotally, autistic pupils reported that teletherapy was 'harder' than in-person therapy due to feeling like they needed to communicate more formally via MS Teams which added an additional mental load to an already demanding situation. Balancing online and in-person methods requires careful consideration – over-reliance on technology may limit the depth of interpersonal connection and nuanced understanding that in-person interactions offer.

Data privacy is another challenge when handling sensitive information. AI applications collect extensive pupil data, raising concerns about storage and sharing despite increased telehealth usage since COVID-19, research on its security and privacy is lacking (Tazi et al., 2024). The Health and Care Professions Council advises professionals to ensure confidentiality is in place by being aware of their surroundings when working remotely. Schools and SaLTs must address concerns around maintaining confidentiality whilst ensuring effective therapy and data use. Joint understanding of privacy expectations and consent must therefore be in place with families and stakeholders.

> ### CHAPTER SUMMARY
>
> This chapter underscores the importance of interprofessional and family-centred collaboration in supporting pupils with SLCN. Effective collaboration integrates the knowledge and skills of various stakeholders, with understanding and consideration of role, setting and/or provision limitations. It highlights the need for a team-oriented approach, addressing systemic barriers and ensuring that collaborative practices are embedded across settings to be effective whilst also remaining family-centred.
>
> Whilst technology, AI and mobile applications offer promising opportunities to enhance collaboration and provision between families, education professionals, colleagues in health/social care and SaLTs, it is important to remember that these opportunities also present challenges in access, privacy and the quality of in-person versus virtual support.
>
> Effective integration of technological tools can enable a more inclusive and responsive educational environment, but it requires careful planning from all parties to ensure equitable and impactful support for all pupils.
>
> Ultimately, successful collaboration requires a focus on the pupil's needs, ongoing professional development and a balance between in-person and digital interactions to achieve positive and long-lasting outcomes for pupils with SLCN.

Further reading/resources

Mathers, A, Botting, N and Moss, R (2024) Collaborative working between speech and language therapists and teaching staff in mainstream UK primary schools: A scoping review. *Child Language Teaching and Therapy.* 40(2): 120–138

- Identification of collaborative strategies in place for UK SaLTs and Educators working together.

RCSLT *Telehealth Guidance* (2022): https://www.rcslt.org/members/delivering-quality-services/telehealth-guidance/ (accessed 24February2025).

- SaLT telehealth guidance which can be used by educators to better understand digital inclusion, consent and information governance.

Suh, H, Dangol, A, Meadan-Kaplansky, H, Miller, C A, and Kientz, J A (2024) *Opportunities and Challenges for AI-Based Support for Speech-Language Pathologists.* Available at. https://doi.org/10.1145/3663384.3663387 (accessed 24 February 2025).

- Identification of opportunities and challenges around digital inclusion, consent and information governance

 References

Cameron, A (2011) Impermeable boundaries? Developments in professional and inter-professional practice. *Journal of Interprofessional Care.* 25(1): 53–58.

Castañer, X and Oliveira, N (2020) Collaboration, coordination, and cooperation among organizations: Establishing the distinctive meanings of these terms through a systematic literature review. *Journal of Management.* 46(6): 965–1001.

Children and Families Act (2014) [online] Available at: https://www.legislation.gov.uk/ukpga/2014/6/contents (accessed 24 February 2025).

Friend, M and Cook, L (2000) *Interactions: Collaboration skills for school professionals.* Third Edition. New York: Longman.

Glover, A, McCormack, J and Smith-Tamaray, M (2015) Collaboration between teachers and speech and language therapists: Services for primary school children with speech, language and communication needs. *Child Language Teaching and Therapy*, 31(3): 363–382.

Gov.UK (2014) SEND code of practice: 0 to 25 years. [online] Available at: https://www.gov.uk/government/publications/send-code-of-practice-0-to-25 (accessed 18 August 2024).

Gov.UK (2023) SEND and alternative provision roadmap. [online] Available at: https://www.gov.uk/government/publications/send-and-alternative-provision-improvement-plan/send-and-alternative-provision-roadmap (accessed 5 October 2024).

Gov.UK (2024) The challenges of teacher recruitment and retention in England. [online] Available at: https://educationinspection.blog.gov.uk/2024/09/17/the-challenges-of-teacher-recruitment-and-retention-in-england/ (accessed 9 November 2024).

Hartas, D (2004) Teacher and speech-language therapist collaboration: Being equal and achieving a common goal? *Child Language Teaching and Therapy,* 20(1): 33–54.

Jeremy, J, Spandagou, I, and Hinitt, J (2024) Teacher-therapist collaboration in inclusive primary schools: A scoping review. *Australian Occupational Therapy Journal*, 71(4): 593–611.

Klatte, I, Bloemen, M, de Groot, A, Mantel, T, Ketelaar, M, and Gerrits, E (2024) Collaborative working in speech and language therapy for children with DLD: What are parents' needs? *International Journal of Language and Communication Disorders*, 59(1): 340–353.

Law, J, Lee, W, Roulstone, S, Wren, Y, Zeng, B, and Lundsay, G (2012) *'What Works': Interventions for Children and Young People with Speech, Language and Communication Needs*. London: Department for Education.

Leinweber, J, Alber, B, Barthel, M, Whillier, A S, Wittmar, S, Borgetto, B and Starke, A, (2023). Technology use in speech and language therapy: digital participation succeeds through acceptance and use of technology. *Frontiers in Communication*, 8, p.1176827.

Mathers, A, Botting, N, and Moss, R (2024) Collaborative working between speech and language therapists and teaching staff in mainstream UK primary schools: A scoping review. *Child Language Teaching and Therapy*, 40(2): 120–138.

Mecrow, C., Beckwith, J., and Klee, T (2010) An exploratory trial of the effectiveness of an enhanced consultative approach to delivering speech and language intervention in schools. *International Journal of Language and Communication Disorders*, 45(3): 354–367.

Nancarrow, S A, Booth, A, Ariss, S, Smith, T, Enderby, P, and Roots, A (2013) Ten principles of good interdisciplinary team-work. *Human Resources for Health*, 11(1): Art. 19.

Ofcom (2023) Communication Market Report 2024: Interactive Data. [online] Available at: https://www.ofcom.org.uk/phones-and-broadband/service-quality/communications-market-report-2024-interactive-data/ (accessed 27 March 2025).

Quigley, D and Smith, M (2021) Achieving effective interprofessional practice between speech and language therapists and teachers: An epistemological perspective. *Child Language Teaching and Therapy*, 38(2): 126–150.

See, B and Gorard, S (2015) The role of parents in young people's education: A critical review of the causal evidence. *Oxford Review of Education*, 41(3): 346–366.

Tazi, F, Dykstra, J, Rajivan, P, and Das, S (2024). "We Have No Security Concerns": Understanding the Privacy-Security Nexus in Telehealth for Audiologists and Speech-Language Pathologists. *Proceedings of the 2024 CHI Conference on Human Factors in Computing Systems* (pp. 1-20). [online] Available at: https://dl.acm.org/doi/10.1145/3613904.3642208 (accessed 27 March 2025).

Wright, J, Stackhouse, J, and Wood, J (2008) Promoting language and literacy skills in the early years: Lessons from interdisciplinary teaching and learning. *Child Language Teaching and Therapy* 24: 155–171.

Conclusion

As we highlighted at the start of this book, '*speech and communication lie at the heart of classroom practice. It is the predominant way in which teachers provide instruction and support to their students and is central to how most students engage with the curriculum*' (Millard and Gaunt, 2018, p. 1). The chapters within this text have illustrated the theory behind the development of communication, the complex but interwoven interplay between communication and education, and how lived experience of speech, language and communication needs has the potential to lock a pupil out of not just the curriculum, but also the myriad of school experiences that allow them to develop into healthy and happy adults.

By this point in the text, you will be very familiar with the term 'speech, language and communication need' or SLCN. It is always vital that while we recognise that we recognise the large number of children with SLCN who will appear with this as their primary need on the SEN Register should each be viewed as an individual with their own experiences, ambitions and strengths.

Anyone working in education will know a child with some kind of SLCN and, realistically, will know many. Perhaps their need is evident and some support is already in place, or perhaps their need is less obvious and they are not yet en route to receiving the help they need. It is our hope that this book has given you some insight into and examples of the ways you can work with these individuals, and tailor the strategies to best support them to achieve their potential.

Speech, language and communication are the primary means we engage with the world around us. It is difficult to underestimate their significance in our daily lives. However, it is certainly easy to take them for granted. As educators, you have the power to effect real change for these learners day in, day out through your practice. Our sincere hope is that this text goes some way towards equipping you with the skills and knowledge to make this change a reality.

Finally, we want to end by expressing how much we value and respect working with each one of you. Indeed, it is through collaboration and teamwork, where we recognise and harness the knowledge and skills of each other, that we will best progress the speech, language and communication skills and outcomes for every child and young person we are privileged to work with.

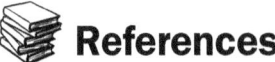# References

Millard, W and Gaunt, A (2018) Speaking up: The importance of oracy in teaching and learning (accessed 4 April 2025).

Index

Pages in *italics* refer to figures and pages in **bold** refer to tables.

ADHD (Attention Deficit Hyperactivity Disorder), prevalence, 32
adulthood preparation, 185–194
  careers/job coaching (face-to-face), 191
  case study (EHCP/autism student), 192–193
  communication (between schools and home), 188
  critical questions, 189, 193
  further education/employment transition, 191–192
  GCSE offer reduction (best interest of student), 193
  GCSE success, 187
  guidance for adaptive teaching, 189
  hands-on learning experiences, 191–193
  interventions available (published), 190
  masking, 191–192
  opportunities to visit new school, 188–189
  primary and secondary setting (key differences), **187–188**
  secondary school transition, 188–189
  secondary school years, 187–189
  self-advocacy and workplace skills, 190–191
  SLCN (persistent), 186
  support services communications, 189
  technology (relationship), 193
  'work experience' programme in school, 192–193
adverse childhood experiences (ACEs), *see* trauma
Affect Autism, 201–202
AI tools, SLCN identification and support, 221
Ainsworth, M D S, 156
Alexander, R, 11, 16
Allen, E, 2
alternative provision (AP), 158–161, 218
'analytic' language processing, *see* Gestalt language processing (GLP)
attachment (positive SEMH), 156
attachment styles, 156, **157**
attention and listening, 23–36
  attention definition, 24–25
  attention development stages (Cooper), 25, **25–26**
  attention main components (Mirsky), 25
  case study (playing video games), 33–34
  challenges (when likely to be present), 31–32

  critical questions, 27–28, 31, 34
  distraction (adolescents), 27
  executive function model (Brown), 27, *27*
  guidance for adaptive teaching, 34–35
  listening, 27–29
  memory and executive functions skills, 26–27
  mental processes, 24
  new media (mobile touchscreen devices (MTSDs)), 32–34
  sensory and environmental factors, 29–31
  SLC sills and their influence, 30–31; *see also* listening
attention capacity
  and trauma, 26
  variation, 26
Auditory Processing Disorder (APD), 28, 200–201
autism
  Affect Autism, 201–202
  attention autism sessions, 132
  behaviourist approaches, 205–206
  behaviours assumed as anxiety reframed as autism, **160**
  behaviours assumed psychosis reframed as autism, **159**
  benefits of adaptations, 134
  case study (Building Together), 207–208
  case study (Pupil A), 132–133
  communication intent and social interaction, 130, 132–134
  critical questions, 133
  double empathy (theory-of-mind problem), 130
  eye contact difficulties, 16
  Gestalt language processing (GLP), 103–104, 134
  Greenspan Floortime Approach®, 134
  neuro-affirming approaches, 206
  neurodiversity movement, 133
  prevalence estimates, 32
  SCERTS approach, 134
  school staffing challenges, 132–133
  SPACE framework, 133–134, *134*, 135
  teletherapy, 222
Ayling, C, and Bamblett, L, 79–90

Bamblett, L
  and Ayling, C, 79–90
  and Capener, N, 92–105
  and Stokes, N, 197–209
behaviour polices (communication-accessible), 170, 173–174, 175
Bercow report (DCSF, 2008), 10
Blanchard, O, and Buchs, A, 46
Blank's levels of questions, 101–102, 120
Bloom, P, and Lahey, M, 128
Bloom's taxonomy, 101
Brackett, M, 61
Branagan, A, et al., 61–62
Brewster, S, 9–21
Bruner, J S, 42
Buchs, A, and Blanchard, O, 46
Burden, J, 57

Capener, N
  and Bamblett, L, 92–105
  and Hopkins, T, 107–123
careers/job coaching (face-to-face), 191
Caribbean creoles, 73
Children and Families Act (2014), pupil and family involvement in decision-making, 215
classroom
  CYP stress and worry, 58
  and e-learning, 58
  and home learning environment, 12
  pedagogy (inclusive), 12–15
  'waves of intervention' model, 12; *see also* emotional regulation (classroom)
Classroom Sensory Environment Assessment, 30
cleft lip and palate, 83
closed questions, teacher talk, 14
cochlear implant, 28–29
cognates, 69
collaborative group work, pedagogy (inclusive), 14
Comic Strip Conversations (Gray), 136, 163, 173
communication intent and social interaction, 124–137
  autism, 130, 132–134
  case study (pupil with autism/global developmental delay), 132–133
  cognitive processing and engagement, 128
  communication functioning (across school day), 135
  communication functions (early), *127*, 135
  communication partners, 135–136
  competence and positive outcomes, 128, 130
  critical questions, 129, 131, 133
  critical thinking (metacognitive activity), 127–128
  expository discourse, 127
  expression of choices and preferences, 128
  guidance for adaptive teaching, 135–136
  intentional communication development, **126**
  language of the curriculum, 127
  opportunities to communicate (creating), 128
  oracy, 128
  pre-intentional and intentional communication, 126

  reasons and intent, 127–128
  rights (laws) CYP to communicate and be heard, 130–131
  social communication, 128–130
  sociolinguistic rules, 130
  specific resources for social communication and interaction, 136
  theory and models, 126–130
Communication Supporting Classroom Observation Tool, 162
concrete, pictorial, abstract (CPA) approach, 42–43
continuous professional development (CPD), 221
Cook, L, and Friend, M, 213
Cooper, J, Moodley, M and Reynell, J, 25–26
Covid-19, emotions and digital engagement, 58
cued articulation, 203–204
  phonics teaching, 204–205
Cushing, I, 14–15

de-escalation strategies, behaviour and exclusion processes, 174–177, *177*
Deafness Research UK, 94
demands and capacities model (Starkweather), 169–170
Department of Education, Behaviour and Attendance policies, 170–171
Derbyshire Sensory Toolkit, 203
Developmental Language Disorder (DLD), 16
  assessment and diagnosis by SaLT, 95
  behavioural difficulties reframed as DLD, **161–162**
  further/higher education accommodations, 192
  interventions available (published), 190
  lifelong condition (understanding), 199
  prevalence, 32, 198
  quiet classrooms, 201
  RADLD (Raising Awareness of DLD) webpage, 96
  and SEMH, 155
dialogic reading, 112–113
dialogic teaching
  pedagogy (inclusive), 11, 14, 16
  'talk'-based pedagogies, 14–15
digital communication, enhancement of school/home communication, 188
digital literacy, 115–116
  CYP relationship with technology, 193
  'ethical digital citizens' (UNESCO), 116; *see also* technology advancements
DLD and Me (Sowerbutts and Finer), 190
Dockrell, J, et al., 199
Doherty, M, et al., 133–134
Donnellan, E, et al., 126

Ecclestone, K, and Hayes, D, 56
education, health and care plans (EHCPs), 192, 207
Education Policy Institute, school exclusion, 171
Elklan-trained school staff, 89
Emmett, A, 141–151, 185–194
emotional dysregulation in schools, 57–60

emotional regulation (classroom), 52–63
  calming strategies, 60
  case study (TA support of stammering child), 59–60
  'deal with feelings', 54
  emotion and communication friendly environments, 61–62
  emotional dysregulation in schools, 53, 57–60
  emotional literacy skills, 53
  enhancing emotional regulation, 59
  inability to regulate seen as poor behaviour, 56–57, 59–60
  language and emotion, 55–57
  and mental health conditions, 56, 58
  'norms', 57
  positive mental health and wellbeing, 53
  process model, 54, 55, 59
  stammering and frustration, 59–60
  supporting skills development, 55
English
  deep orthographic language, 110
  grapheme to phoneme correspondence (GPC), 110
  homophones, 110
  morphological training/instruction, 110
  non-standard dialects debate, 16, 73
  semantics, 110
English as an additional language (EAL), increasing in school population, 16
English for speakers of other languages (ESOL), parents' hub, 18
Equality Act (2010)
  reasonable adjustments duty, 172–173, 190
  stammer support for CYP, 147
Equals Curriculum, 206
executive function model (Brown), 27, 27
expository writing, 114–115

Friend, M, and Cook, L, 213
further/higher education
  accommodations for DLD, 192
  masking and identification of SLCN, 191–192

Garćia, O, and Wei, L, 73
Gaunt, A., and Millard, W, 1
Gestalt language processing (GLP), 103–104
  autism, 103, 134
  interventions, 104
  repeated phrases, 103
Glasby, J, et al., 199
glue ear, 31, 94–95
Google Translate, 221
Google Workspace, 221
Graves, M F, 97
Grehan, H, 29
Grice, H P, 130
Gross, J, 12, 19

hands-on learning experiences, 191–193
Hayes, C, 28

Hayes, D, and Ecclestone, K, 56
Health and Care Professions Council, 223
hearing difficulties
  auditory environment in classroom, 94
  classroom strategies, 94–95
  glue ear (case study), 94–95
  physical hearing impairment, 29
Hobson, H, et al., 55
Hopkins, T, 39–49
  and Capener, N, 107–123
Hutchins, T L, et al., 103

inclusive environments, 197–209
  accessible environment, 200–202
  accessible pedagogies, 199
  background noise difficulties, 200–201
  capability and understanding of SLCN (Glasby study), 198–199
  case study (Building Together), 206
  communication friendly classrooms, 202
  critical questions, 205, 208
  dysregulation and disruption, 200
  guidance for adaptive planning, 203
  inclusion and raising academic standards (differing agendas), 199
  inclusive classroom (barriers), 200
  language screening (early years), 205
  mainstream classroom inclusive practice (all CYP), 199
  neurodiversity debate, 205–206
  quiet classrooms, 201
  reasonable adjustments duty, 201
  seating plan, 201
  SEND Code of Practice, 199
  SEND crisis in UK schools, 198
  SEND teaching within mainstream class (challenge), 202
  specific pedagogical approaches, 203–205
  targeted interventions, 207
  uniform changes, 201
  universal approaches, 203, **204**
initial teacher training (ITT), core content framework, 1–2
interprofessional and collaborative working, 211–224
  case studies, 119–120, 217–218, 220, 222
  collaborative partners, 213
  common goals, 214
  critical questions, 214
  evaluating the impact of collaborative practices, 220–221
  family-centred collaboration, 215–216
  group work in a nursery setting (case study), 219
  health services and education, 213
  implementation challenges, 216
  Microsoft SharePoint (case study), 222
  one-to-one sixth form supported internships (case study), 220
  online and in-person methods (balancing), 222–223
  opportunities available, 216–221

parents feeling of disempowerment, 216
reviews of in UK primary schools, 215
SaLT support essential, 216
skills (complementary transfer), 215
systemic barriers, 215
TAs work on SaLT interventions/views on collaborations, 215
teacher and SaLT co-teaching (case study), 119–120
teamwork (integral to schools and service delivery), 212
technology advancements, 221–223
theories and principles, 214
whole class emotional regulation AP (case study), 218
whole school task plans (case study), 217
workforce pressures, 214–215

Jolly Phonics, 204–205
judgment on participation, impairment, anxiety, or behaviour, 15, 31

knowledge
  co-construct, 14
  interaction as essential to acquiring and understanding, 12
Knowler, H, 52–63
  and Westwood, C, 167–180

Lahey, M, and Bloom, P, 128
Lambert, M, and Rozsahegyi, T, 10, 199
Lancastle, D, et al., 57
language acquisition, interactionist perspectives, 45
Language for Behaviour and Emotions (Branagan, Cross and Parsons), 61–62, 136, 189
language screening (early years), 205
language (understanding and using), 92–105
  assessment and diagnosis by SaLT, 95
  Bloom's taxonomy mapped to Blank's levels, *101*
  'bottom-up' processes, 98
  case study (glue ear), 94–95
  challenges (presentation), 95–102
  challenges with sentence building/narrative skills, **98**
  cognitive effort and stress, 102
  colour coding and use of symbols, *99*
  complex language, 101–102
  CPY can fool adults with learnt format responses, 102
  critical questions, 95
  hearing difficulties, 94–95
  'higher-level' language skills, 101–102
  language (what is), 93–94
  sentence building and narrative, 97–99
  spoken language and academic progress, 93
  strategies for 'higher-level' language, *102*
  strategies for sentence building/narrative skills, 99
  teacher's instructions (understanding), 93
  'top-down' processes, 97, 101
  verbal and written communication, 94
  vocabulary, 96–97; *see also* Gestalt language processing (GLP)

Law, J, et al., 216–217
league tables, and exclusion, 170–171
Lego-based therapy, 206
  case study (Building Together), 207–208
Li, P, 67
listening
  active, 29
  active process, 28–29
  auditory processing difficulties, 28
  critical questions, 27–28
  effective (tips for), 35
  selective, 29
  skills can be taught, 28
  switch costs, 28
  thoughtful, 29
  types, 29
Listening skills-BBC Teach, 35
literacy and language, 107–123
  assessments for dyslexia or SLCN, 117
  case study (partnership teacher and SaLT co-teaching), 119–120
  common errors spoken/written, 115
  critical questions, 109, 120
  digital literacy, 115–116
  expository writing, 114–115
  grapheme to phoneme correspondence (GPC), 110
  guidance for adaptive planning, 117
  learning to read and spell, 110
  literacy as biologically secondary knowledge, 109
  'literacy' term, 108–109
  novel words/non-words decoding, 110
  phonological awareness, 110
  reading comprehension, 111–114, 118
  and SaLTs, 109–110, 119–120
  SEND CYP and exam results with SaLT co-teaching, 119–120
  SLCN prevalence, 109
  spelling irregular words, 110
  support strategies, **118–119**
  'top-down' processes, 109

Makaton signs, 74, 99
mapping theory, 41
masking, and further education, 191–192
Maslow's Hierarchy of Needs, 30, 200, *201*
Mayer, R E, 58
McGregor, K K, 170
McLachlan, H, 102
means, reasons and opportunities model (Money and Thurman), 127–128, *129*
'meltdowns', 192–193
memory
  and executive function skills, 26–27
  long-term memory, 41
  semantic memory network, 41
  storage (hierarchal manner), 41
Memory Magic (Booth), 18
mental health conditions, and SLCN, 56, 58

Microsoft SharePoint, 221
  collaborative practices case study, 222
Millard, W, and Gaunt, A., 1
Miller, A D, 27
Milton, D, 130
Mirsky, A F, 25
Money, D, and Thurman, S, 127
Moodley, M, Cooper, J and Reynell, J, 25–26
motor conditions, 16
Moxam, C, 110
multilingualism, 65–75
  additional language after preschool, 68
  assessing language development, 71–72
  assessment and discussions with family, 72, 86
  assessment required indicators for (SLCN), **74–75**
  assessment tools, 71–72, 86
  benefits of, 73
  bilingual or dual language learners, 66
  case study (nursey teacher), 74
  code-switching, 71
  competence in each language, 69
  critical questions, 69, 74
  culturally specific concepts, 72
  emergent multilingual (EM), 66, 69–71
  examples of language exposure, **67–68**
  extent in UK, 66
  grammatical differences (EMs), 71
  'heritage language' (HL), 66, 69–70, 72, 74
  language development in multilingual CYP, 69–71
  language learning and context, 69
  multilingualism (term), 66
  non-standard dialects debate, 73
  sequential language acquisition, 68–69
  'silent period', 70
  simultaneous language acquisition, 67–68
  and SLCN, 72
  SLCN not caused by, 73, 81, 85
  support guidance, 70
  supporting development of multilingual CYP, 72–73
  translanguaging, 73
Murphy, A, and Philpotts, S, 211–224

National Curriculum
  child's age and ZPD, 200
  Equals Curriculum, 206
  insufficient guidance, 11
  presentational talk/Standard English models, 15
  removal of speaking and listening, 17
National Deaf Children's Society, 94
Ne'eman, A, 205
neurodiversity debate, 205–206
  behaviourist approaches, 205–206
  naturalistic, interest-driven group working opportunities, 206
  neuro-affirming approaches, 206
  'right' way to educate cohorts, 205
  Superflex, 206
  Zones of Regulation, 206

neurodiversity movement
  autism, 133
  difference vs deficit, 146–147
new media (mobile touchscreen devices (MTSDs)), attention and listening, 32–34
non-standard dialects, 16, 73

Oakshott-Marston, T, and Westwood, C, 153–164
Ofsted (2024) inspection framework, 58
oracy
  clarity of speech, 13
  increasing profile, 13
  pedagogy (inclusive), 11, 13–14
  skills development, 2, 128
  and social justice, 2
  speaking/listening modalities of communication, 14
  third component, 13
  underplay of listening (rebalance), 13
  "vague term", 128
Oracy Benchmarks (Voice21, 2020), 13
Oracy Education Commission, report (2024), 13, 16
Oracy Framework (2021), 13, 15, 128

Passey, J, 86–87, 203
pedagogy (inclusive), 9–21
  approach (same) to all learners, 11
  case study (SLCN and learners over five), 17–18
  classroom context, 12–15
  collaborative group work, 14
  communication diversity (valuing), 15
  critical questions, 10, 15, 18
  dialogic teaching, 11, 14, 16
  inclusive environments, 203–205
  information and resources for educators, 19–20
  knowledge (co-construct), 14
  management of education and curriculum, 11
  oracy, 11, 13–14
  SLCN identification and assessment, 16
  'talk'-based pedagogies, 14–15
  targeted and specialist intervention, 16–17
  teachers developing own expertise, 18
peek-a boo, 45
person-centred care, and speech and language therapy (SLT), 2
Philpotts, S, and Murphy, A, 211–224
phonics teaching, cued articulation, 204–205
physical hearing impairment, 29
Piaget, J, 44
play and conceptual development, 39–49
  abstract concepts, 42, 45
  case study (Shakespeare role play), 46–47
  concept understanding (fully) debate, 48
  conceptual understanding (definition), 40
  concrete, pictorial, abstract (CPA) approach, 42–43
  critical questions, 43, 47
  culturally specific concepts, 45
  emotion concepts, 42
  guidance for adaptive teaching, 48–49

human rights (UN) to play opportunities, 43–44
joint attentive play, 45–46
and memory, 41
Montessori approach, 44
Piagetian theory, 44
play (benefits), 43
play (no standard definition), 43
play types, 43
promoting play, 44
prototypes (symbolic), 41–42
referents, 40–41
role play, 46–47
running commentary, 46
scaffold opportunities, 40–41
social side of play, 45–46
socio-cultural context, 45
symbolism (importance), 43–44
target concept teaching guidance, 48–49
teaching concepts, 42
theoretical explanations (concept development), 41–43
toys and resources, 44
zone of proximal development (ZPD), 41–42
Pollard, A, 14
primary impairment
  referrals to external specialist services, 17
  and SLCN, 17
psycho-social development, and SLCN, 56
pupils, disadvantaged backgrounds and additional needs, 1

Quality First Teaching (QFT), 199–200, 203

reading comprehension, 111–114
  critical questions, 114
  dialogic reading, 112–113
  heuristic for thinking about reading comprehension (Snow), 112, *112*
  'learned helplessness' (motivation to read), 113–114
  low confidence (support for CYP), 113–114
  psycholinguistic perspectives, 111–112
  reading as social practice, 112–113
  simple view of reading, 111, *111*
  socio-cultural norms and practices, 112
  support strategies, 118
Reynell, J, Cooper, J and Moodley, M, 25–26
Richards, H, 23–36, 124–137
Rights of the Child (UNCRC), 130
Ripley, K, and Yuill, N, 53
role play, 18, 46–47
  debriefing session, 46
  Shakespeare (case study), 46–47
Royal College of Speech and Language Therapists (RCSLT)
  Mind Your Words / The Box training, 174
  SLCN assessment, 169
Rozsahegyi, T, and Lambert, M, 11, 199
RULER method (Brackett), 61
Rutter, M, 56

Salamanca Statement (UNESCO), 198
school exclusion process, 167–180
  behaviour polices (communication-accessible), 170, 173–174, *175*
  behavioural difficulties and undiagnosed SLCN, 168
  case studies, 172–173, 178–179
  critical questions, 170, 178
  critical reflection, 171
  de-escalation strategies, 174–177, *177*
  demands and capacities model (Starkweather), 169–170
  disciplinary reasons (vague), 169
  exclusion prevalence, 169
  fixed term (a suspension), 169
  headteacher guidance DfE (2024), 169
  informal and unlawful exclusion, 170–171
  league tables, 170–171
  legal actions and hidden SLCN (link), **172**
  mislabelling of CYP with SLCN and SEMH as 'naughty', 170
  multi-step instruction difficulties and SaLT assessment, 178
  permanent (removal from school setting), 169
  persistent disruptive behaviour, 168, 178
  primary to secondary school demands, 169–170
  safe exit strategies, 178
  SaLT assessments, 178–179
  school-to-prison pipeline, 170
  SLCN assessment, 169
  strategies for support (reflective checklist), **173–174**
  swearing in class, 178
  training (identifying and support for SLCN), 174
  understanding (no) of 'how?' and 'why?' questions SaLT assessments, 179
  verbal based interventions and reasonable adjustments, 172–173
  verbal competence (pupils and families involved), 171
school level, SEN budget, 18
'school ready' learners, 56
SEND Code of Practice, 130–131, 199
  'assess, plan, do, review' (APDR) cycles, 221
  pupil and family involvement in decision-making, 215
sensorineural hearing impairment, 29
sensory environment, suitable provision, 30
sensory processing difficulties, 29–30
Sensory Processing Disorder (SPD), prevalence, 200
Snell, J, 15
Snow, P C, 108, 112
Social and Emotional Aspects of Learning (SEAL), 56
social and emotional learning (SEL) programmes, 56
social constructivist theory or learning, 11–12
social disadvantage, and SLCN, 12, 14–15
social, emotional and mental health (SEMH) needs, 2–3, 153–164
  alternative provision (AP), 158–161
  attachment (positive SEMH), 156, **157**
  behavioural difficulties reframed as DLD, **161–162**

behaviours assumed as anxiety reframed as autism, **160**
behaviours assumed psychosis reframed as autism, **159**
case study (AP for DLD CYP), 161–162
case study (AP for situationally mute CYP), 159–160
critical questions, 157
Developmental Language Disorder (DLD), 155
language adaptation, 162
multi-agency differential diagnosis, 159
prevalence, 154
primary to secondary school, 169–170
pupil referral unit (PRU), 159
referral thresholds, 155
reframing SEMH as SLCN, 158–159
relationship SLCN and SEMH, 154–157
school exclusion process, 169
SLCN screening, 158
social skills inclusivity, 163
strategies for adaptive planning, 162–163
trauma (adverse childhood experiences (ACEs)), 156, **156**
unmet needs and negative life chances, 155
visual cues, 162, **163**
social justice, and oracy skills development, 2
social scripts, 206
Social Stories (Gray), 136
speech, 79–90
atypical speech error patterns, **84–85**
case study (mainstream primary, SSD and ADHD), 88–89
critical questions, 89
CYP who speak multiple languages debate, 85–86
CYP with unclear speech (supporting), 86–89
development progression and speech of younger children, 82
multilingualism, 81, 85–86
phonological awareness, 80, 87, 89
referrals to SLT, 85
speech definition, 80
Speech Sound Disorder (SSD), 80, 83–85
typical development of speech sounds, 81–83
typical speech error patterns, **82–83**; see also multilingualism
speech and language development delays, 1
speech and language therapists (SaLTs)
caseloads, 214
essential support in educational settings, 216
and literacy, 109–110, 119–120
stammer referrals, 150
speech and learning therapy (SLT)
and person-centred care, 2
role of teaching assistant, 17
speech, language and communication needs (SLCN)
adverse childhood experiences (ACEs), 156, **156**
assessment required indicators for multilingual CYP, **74–75**
catch-all term, 12–13

identification and assessment, 16
increasing, 1, 10
masking and identification as adults, 191–192
and mental health conditions, 56, 58
multilingualism (not caused by), 73, 81, 85
poor funding/teachers developing own expertise, 18
prevalence, 109, 226
and psycho-social development, 56
reframing SEMH as SLCN, 158–159
relationship SLCN and SEMH, 154–157
risk of social and emotional difficulties, 56
screening in CYP with SEMH, 158
stammer co-occurring, 146
speech, language and communication (SLC), skill and mental processes, 24
Speech Sound Disorder (SSD), 80, 83–85
articulation, 83
atypical speech error patterns, **84–85**
case study (mainstream primary, SSD and ADHD), 88–89
critical questions, 89
CYP with unclear speech (supporting), 86–89
emphasising sounds in speech (teacher), 86
home-school communication book, 87
modelling accurate speech, 86
motor speech disorders, 84
other terms for, 83
peer's reactions, 87
phonological awareness, 87, 89
phonology, 84
prevalence, 198
reasonable adjustments, 87
relationships, 88–89
self-esteem, 86
SLT services involvement, 88–89
speech targets work, 87
TA as familiar listener, 88
using cued articulation in phonics, 86–87
speech sounds, typical and atypical, 2
stammer, 16
stammer (enabling communication), 141–151
anxiety and negative self-views, 145
awareness (CYP), 148
case study (one-to-one assessment), 149–150
causes, 143
communication difference in the flow of speech, 142, 146
coping strategies, 150
covert stammering, 144
critical questions, 144, 150
difference vs deficit (neurodiversity movement), 146–147
emotions as trigger, 143
fear of negative reactions, 144
genetic influence, 143
guidance for adaptive teaching, 147–149
iceberg analogy, *145*
impact of, 145

instanced for every talker (nervous or tired), 142
myths and realities, 144, 146
neurodevelopment conditions (CYP with), 146
neurological (brain-based), 143
prevalence, 142
psychogenic cause, 143
referral to SaLT, 150
'secondary' or 'concomitant' behaviours, 142
SLCN co-occurring, 146
social model of disability, 146–147
special educational needs (other), 146
stigma, 146
support for CYP (legal requirement), 147
Stokes, N, and Bamblett, L, 197–209
Stringer, H, 87
stuttering, see stammer
Suphi, A, 65–75
swearing in class, school exclusion process, 178
switch costs, 28

Talk for Work ('Speech and Language UK'), 190
Talkabout Series (Kelly), 136, 163
Talking Mats, 173
teacher sensory screening, 201–202
teacher talk, closed questions, 14
teaching assistant (TA)
   interprofessional and collaborative working, 215
   role in SLT, 17
technology advancements
   AI tools, 221
   communication aids, 221
   data privacy, 223
   digital divide, 222
   document collaboration, 221
   ethical challenges, 222–223
   interprofessional and collaborative working, 221–223
   teletherapy, 222
   tracking pupils progress, 221
   video conferencing, 221
telehealth usage, security and privacy, 223
teletherapy, 222
Thurman, S, and Money, D, 127
Time to Talk, 89
trauma
   adverse childhood experiences (ACEs), 156
   and attention capacity, 26
   prevalence, 32
   and SLCN, 156, **156**
   traumatic stress, 32

uniform changes, 201

video conferencing, 221
vocabulary, 96–97
   academic success in core subjects, 96
   effective teaching, 97
   established strategies and considerations, 97
   expressive, 96
   receptive, 96
   target words, 96
   three tiers examples, **96**, 97
voice (agency and views), rights (laws) CYP to communicate and be heard, 130–131
Vygotsky, L S, 12, 44, 200

waves of intervention model, 12, 200
Wei, L, and Garćia, O, 73
wellbeing, social and emotional, 1, 53; see also emotional regulation (classroom)
Westwood, C
   and Knowler, H, 167–180
   and Oakshott-Marston, T, 153–164
Widgit vocabulary mats, 207
Window of Tolerance theory, 60
word maps, 120

Yip, V, 67
Yuill, N, and Ripley, K, 53

zone of proximal development (ZPD), 41–42
   and National Curriculum, 200

For Product Safety Concerns and Information please contact our EU
representative GPSR@taylorandfrancis.com
Taylor & Francis Verlag GmbH, Kaufingerstraße 24, 80331 München, Germany

www.ingramcontent.com/pod-product-compliance
Lightning Source LLC
Chambersburg PA
CBHW080837230426
43665CB00021B/2861